IT'S NOT JUST ABOUT

THE SUGAR

LIVING WITH DIABETES

Marie A.C. Cortez, LCSW

Dedication

To the boys in my life:

Hernán, Sr.; Hernán, Jr. and Marco Antonio

Table of Contents

A Word From the Author

Trial 10,000+: The approximate number of days I have lived with type 1 diabetes. It is also the number of days I have tried to make good choices in my eating habits and in how I choose to treat my diabetes. While my eating habits today are not atrocious like they were twenty-five plus years ago, I still struggle every day to make the right choices.

The first time I heard the words, "Marie…you are diabetic, you need insulin for the rest of your life," it felt like a death sentence. After all, all I knew about diabetes was in regard to people needing amputations, going blind, and needing dialysis. The diagnosis of diabetes did not seem hopeful at that time. To this day, it amazes me that diabetes continues to be such a mystery to many. As long as I have lived with my diabetes (30+ years), I still have people close to me ask, "What type of diabetes do you have? Is that the bad one?" I wonder why diabetes still seems so mysterious, or does society just choose to play ignorant? Or am I just not tolerant enough?

Before I go on, I want to touch base on the topic of diabetic vs. PWD (Person With Diabetes[1]). The term PWD was not around at the time of my diagnosis. I was told I was now a diabetic and for the longest time, I have considered myself a diabetic or, as I tell my husband and others, "*I am extra special, I am # 1.*" It's how I hope they will remember that I am type 1 and not type 2. It's only been very recently that I learned about the PWD term. I don't use this term often to describe myself when talking about my diabetes, but please know this is *my* situation. I feel comfortable saying I am a type 1 diabetic. As a mental health provider, I understand the power that words have. Labels can be good or bad, they can heal or hurt. If you have been diagnosed with diabetes, use the term that feels good for you. If you know of someone that has diabetes, ask them how they identify with their diabetes. They will be delighted that you have taken the time to be thoughtful. In this book, I will use the terms **PWD** (Person With Diabetes) and **T1D** as a shortcut for type 1 diabetes and **T2D** as a shortcut for type 2 diabetes. Please know that "PWD" includes both those with type 1 and those with type 2.

Thanks to science, biomedical engineering, and those who have a vision of a better life for those with diabetes, the words I heard when I was given my diagnosis no longer feel like a death sentence. Or at least not one that is without hope. Given all the technology that exists today for those living with type 1 diabetes, living with diabetes can feel very motivating, exciting, and innovative. Okay, who am I kidding? Not exactly! Living with diabetes is HELL. It's difficult, challenging, exhausting, and unpredictable. But on a "good day",

today's technology makes me feel hopeful. **<u>Every day</u>**
<u>of my life is a trial!</u>

This book is coming from a patient's perspective.
It is also about how type 1 diabetes impacts the human
body that deals with it on a day-to-day basis, twenty-four
hours a day, 365/366 days a year, for the rest of one's
life! And yes, diabetes affects the entire body in many
ways. Often, it can be visible to the eye; other times, not
so much. That patient is me. Besides being a patient, I
am a licensed clinical social worker and I am very
familiar with human struggles. For everyone that shares
my diagnosis, T1D is a human struggle, a very unique
struggle. For everyone that has the diagnosis of type 2,
this book can benefit you as well.

According to an article[2] on diabetesdaily.com,
the disease of "diabetes" as we refer to it today was

discovered in ancient times before Christ, but it was not until 1922 when the first human patient received insulin treatment. And here we are today, the year 2022, and diabetes still remains without a cure. The research, the understanding of diabetes and its treatments has come a LONG WAY; however, if you are a PWD or if you live with someone that is and you see their daily struggles, you know it is a difficult road.

My hopes for this book and for its readers are as follows:

If you are T1D, T2D, or a PWD:
- I hope you realize you are NOT alone!
- I hope you realize that today's technology can be empowering. It can bring some relief to the struggle and help you manage your treatment plan.
- I hope you realize what a critical role you can play not only in your personal treatment, but also in our society as an educator and advocate.

If you are not a PWD:

- I hope you come to understand diabetes and realize that it can happen to anyone.

If you are a healthcare professional:

- I hope this book helps you to view diabetes from the patient's perspective. Please, continue to be kind, tolerant, understanding and empathetic. Trust me, we are trying!

Finally, a PWD or not, I hope you get to pass on everything you learn in this book and share it with the world.

In addition, here are some additional and helpful links for learning about diabetes:

http://www.diabetes.org/living-with-diabetes/complications/mental-health/depression.html

http://www.cdc.gov/diabetes/consumer/learn.htm

http://www.niaid.nih.gov/topics/immuneSystem/Pages/

disorders.aspx

http://www.bam.gov/sub_yourbody/yourbody_diabetes

_questions.html#6

http://www.niaid.nih.gov/Pages/default.aspx

Marie A.C. Cortez
Licensed Clinical Social Worker/Author

Chapter I: The Big News

It was December 1991, a cold winter and the season I struggle with the most because I love warm weather. I was on vacation about 8 hours away from home when I returned a call from the doctor I had seen at the walk-in clinic before leaving for my vacation. I was hoping to get a quick and easy answer as to why I was so thirsty all the time, exhausted, and having to use the bathroom more than ever in my life. Could I be pregnant? Even though I was in a serious relationship at the time, I sure wasn't ready to be a mom, but the thought was intriguing and exciting.

The doctor on the other end of the phone line was hundreds of miles away. "Your blood work was abnormal in some areas. It's not mono and you are not anemic." You see, when I first went to the doctor's office, I told the doctor that I was sure I had mononucleosis or that I was anemic. I had a history of being anemic as a child, so I was sure that was the case here. I was falling asleep behind the wheel, there was not a second that I was not feeling exhausted. I felt and looked like hell, having lost about 12 pounds in about a year and I was not big to begin with. I just did not feel right.

The doctor continues, "We are concerned about your glucose level and we need to have a follow up appointment with you. When can you come back to the clinic?" Well, there goes my vacation, I said to myself. Luckily it was a short vacation and I would be home in a few days. After scheduling my next appointment, I tell the doctor, "I've been so thirsty and I keep drinking soda and going to the bathroom." The doctor instructs me to stay away from soda and high fructose drinks, and to only drink water when I am feeling thirsty. At this time in my life, I was not a fan of drinking water and I must sadly admit that it took years, I mean *years*, before I finally realized how beneficial and essential drinking water is to the human body.

Back at home a few days later, I return to the doctor's office and the news arrives: "I'm afraid you are diabetic," the doctor announces. I felt a sharp pain go through my chest! Everything I knew about diabetes was that people had their legs amputated, people died from diabetes, and PWDs are not supposed to eat candy or sugar. I almost cried at the doctor's office but I controlled myself. Even though I was relieved that I was not pregnant, pregnancy sounded like a much more doable task and like a much more exciting adventure compared to the cards that life had just dealt me. Looking back, I truly wonder how long I might have been living with diabetes and just did not know it.

The doctor tells me that I have type 2 diabetes (yes, this is not a typo, please keep reading) and, in addition to changing the way I eat, I will also have to take some pills. When I get home, the only one there is my loyal, loving yellow labrador retriever, Shabba (may her soul rest in peace!) I share my news with her and break down in tears. She tries to console me by licking my tears away. I kept seeing images of what I knew about diabetes, what diabetes looked like to me. I remembered my mom's uncle, my great-uncle, whom I had only met once or twice as a child. I remembered how obese he was and how unhealthy he looked. I remembered when I asked my mom why he looked that way, she simply said, "Oh, he has diabetes." I remembered a friend of the family who lived with diabetes and was also obese. At this time in my life, I was thin, weighing about 118 pounds at 5 foot, ¾ inches tall, but there I was, diagnosed with type 2 diabetes. It didn't make sense to me, I didn't fit the mold of what I knew at the time about diabetes.

When thinking about treating diabetes, I remembered how people talked about insulin injections and one of the scariest consequences of untreated diabetes-*amputations*! I could not get that image of my mind and kept thinking, "People with diabetes lose their legs." For whatever reason, they didn't seem to lose other things but I remembered they could lose their legs or feet because their diabetes gave them gangrene. In a nutshell, I knew that diabetes could kill me and I was terrified. I was only 22 years old at the time.

On a lighter note, I thought of how much I loved junk food- the French fries, the meat, the rice, and candy. Oh yes, candy! If I had a weakness at that time in my life, it was my passion for junk food. As I mentioned, I was very, very thin at the time of my diagnosis. Back then, I never had the need to make a connection between unhealthy foods and weight gain. It never mattered how I ate, weight gain was not a problem for me. As a matter of fact, back then, I wished I was heavier. Yes, you read that correctly. I was a twig back then and I wished I had meat on my bones (be careful what you wish for.)

At the time of my diagnosis, my eating habits were atrocious. My idea of eating vegetables meant heating up a can of corn. Candy? If you saw how I ate candy, you would have thought I was a five year old. Oh, did I love candy, especially chocolate. I would constantly skip meals, eat candy and ice cream as a meal, and vegetables and salads were never, ever part of my diet. When I did eat or cook a meal, these consisted of some of the following food items: white rice, potatoes, white bread, pasta, meat (mostly red meats), eggs (lots of them) and fried plantains, both green and sweet. There was very little variety in my food choices. Mind you, I was an adult, young, but an adult at this point in my life. I was a very, very picky adult when it came to food.

What I didn't know at the time of my diagnosis was that it wasn't just my eating habits that needed to change, it was much more than that. I didn't know then that:

- My relationship with food needed to change
- My diabetes was going to become my full-time job
- My life would forever, from the point of diagnosis, revolve around my diabetes

You see, I had a very interesting relationship with food. Not only did I have a very limited selection of foods that I liked, a limited selection that was also unhealthy, but I came to have this relationship with food where I saw it as a source of comfort, not a source of fuel. Back then, if you were to ask me, "As a child, how did you know that your father loved you," my response would have been, "He cooks for me, whatever dish I want." If you were to ask me, "What does your mom love to do for you," I would say, "She wants to cook for me." As a parent myself, I have memories of enjoying certain activities with my boys where food played a big role: baking birthday cakes, watching television and eating peanut butter out of the jar, watching movies and munching on popcorn or Tootsie Roll Pops. Most humans have made emotional connections with food and I was no exception, but when I was diagnosed with diabetes, I realized that food needed to play a different role in my life. Here I am years later and I confess that this is no easy task.

As the years have passed, I have come to learn that the older I get, the more changes I have to make. For example, the one cup of white rice that my 25-year-old body accepted is not being as easily accepted by my body in its 50's. As I age with my diabetes, I've learned that my body has become very sensitive to simple carbohydrates. You know, those carbohydrates that can be so addicting like French fries, white rice, bagels, and pretty much any kind of bread.

I can honestly say that my relationship with food has been my biggest struggle in the last twenty years. Think of all the people that you know. How many of those individuals don't like food? The point is not whether they like healthy or unhealthy foods. The point is that most human beings LOVE TO EAT! You see, the other side of the coin that I didn't know at the time of the diagnosis was the fact that:

Food would eventually become my worst enemy, yet it would also be the key to my survival.

This is a hard balance to accomplish and maintain on a day-to-day basis.

Going back to that cold December: as I moped in my sadness for days, weeks, and months, the thought that I could never, ever again have chocolate and candy (or so I thought) was torture. It was very hard for me to accept my diagnosis. I must admit that it took years, that's right, years for me to not only accept my diabetes but also for me to realize the seriousness of my diagnosis. It took a long time for me to realize that if I wanted to live a fulfilling, long and healthy life, I really needed to make some serious and permanent changes in my actions and in my eating habits. This became a greater reality a year later when I found out that my diagnosis as a type 2 diabetic was a medical error, I was actually type 1. Based on my age, weight, and how sick I was initially, I was clearly misdiagnosed the first time around.

I now invite you to follow me on my journey as I live with type 1 diabetes as a woman, wife, working mother, friend, sister, a person with diabetes. This journey has been quite the ride for me. As you follow me on this journey, I hope you enjoy it and most importantly, I hope you find comfort and support in learning how unique type 1 diabetes can be. I also hope that you will have a clearer understanding of type 1 diabetes and what it looks like once you are done with this book.

Chapter II: The Big Picture

In this book, I will take you on **my journey** and my experience as a person living with T1D; but before I do that, I want to talk a little about type 1 diabetes. When someone is diagnosed with diabetes, there are three possible diagnoses but first, let's look at the BIG PICTURE!

Please remember, I am not a doctor or a scientist, but I am fascinated by science. I am a believer that science explains it all but we don't always ask the right questions and we aren't always motivated to understand the mechanics of our illnesses or health issues. I feel it is important for me to dig a little bit deeper into the science of the human body and type 1 diabetes before we move on to my own experience.

The pancreas produces two hormones, insulin and glucagon. Let us imagine a person who isn't living with diabetes eats a meal. The body's physical process is to absorb the sugar from that meal, causing the glucose levels in their bloodstream to rise. The **beta cells** in the pancreas will sense this and will automatically release insulin into the bloodstream. This insulin allows the cells all over the body to take up and absorb the glucose, which is then either used for energy or stored in the liver for later use. Either way, the individual ends up with blood glucose levels in the proper range because things are properly functioning. According to the American Diabetes Association, normal levels/numbers are as follows: before any meal, one should have a blood glucose of 80-130 mg/dl; and one to two hours after a meal, one should have a blood glucose below 180[3].

How about the other hormone created by the pancreas, glucagon? Keep in mind our bodies are like machines and they function perfectly (most of the time). If the blood glucose levels go too low in a person that does not have diabetes, the **alpha cells** in the pancreas release glucagon into the bloodstream. This process tells the liver to release the stored glucose, stabilizing the glucose levels and returning them to normal.

Insulin and glucagon are responsible for regulating blood glucose levels in our bodies. Having diabetes causes hyperglycemia, a fancy way of saying there are unhealthy elevated blood glucose levels in the bloodstream. Believe it or not, type 1 diabetes is considered an uncommon disease. According to the CDC[4], it affects about 5 to 10% of people. Type 1 diabetes falls under a huge umbrella called autoimmune diseases[5]. An autoimmune disease occurs when a person's immune system attacks his/her body by mistake. Yes, you read correctly, our bodies can attack us. The immune system's role is to protect us from germs like bacteria and viruses. When our autoimmune system detects these strange visitors in our bodies, it sends out fighter cells to attack them. In a perfect scenario, our immune system can differentiate between foreign cells and our own cells; however, in an autoimmune disease, the immune system mistakes a part of the body, like the joints, skin, pancreas, or other parts, as foreign. When this happens, the autoimmune system sends out proteins called autoantibodies and attacks healthy cells or organs. In type 1 diabetes, the immune system antibodies attack and permanently destroy the insulin-producing cells (the beta cells) in the pancreas. Because the body can no longer produce insulin, someone living with type 1 diabetes will be required to take insulin for life in order to survive. Believe me, we need insulin more than anything else. I have fasted before needing a medical procedure or a surgery and have been fine; however, I cannot skip my insulin and be okay. I will definitely have to adjust the amount of insulin I take (because of the fasting); but my body still needs insulin.

Regardless of whether you are a woman or a man, or you identify as lesbian, gay, bisexual, transgender, queer, questioning, intersex, pansexual, two-spirit (2S), androgynous, or asexual, please know that diabetes does not discriminate; it can affect anyone. So how did my type 1 diabetes occur? At some point in my early twenties, there was a destruction of my pancreas beta cells and my body was no longer able to produce insulin, which caused my blood glucose levels to be extremely high. What caused the destruction? Well, experts[6] say that I was born with a genetic predisposition or a susceptibility to this disease I was not born with, and an environmental trigger caused my immune system antibodies to attack and destroy the insulin-producing cells (the beta cells) in my pancreas.

Here is a brief look into the two other diagnoses (there are theories, studies, research, etc. of other types of diabetes other than the three discussed in this book, but I'm not going to discuss them here[7]):

1.   Type 2 diabetes - This type of diabetes occurs when either the pancreas fails to produce enough insulin or the insulin is not being properly used by the body. Some people diagnosed with this kind of diabetes can manage it with regular exercise, healthy eating, and weight maintenance. These individuals may also use oral medications and/or insulin injections to manage their diabetes. Think of it as having a lazy pancreas that needs YOUR help.[8]

2.   Gestational diabetes- This diagnosis is only given to pregnant people. It is given when the body is not able to make and use all the insulin it needs for pregnancy. This diagnosis usually only lasts through the pregnancy. Research[9] has shown, however, that people who are

diagnosed with gestational diabetes are more likely to develop type 2 diabetes down the road.

If one is diagnosed with type 2 diabetes, the ride and experience are vastly different from that of a type 1 diagnosis. If these individuals change their diet, increase their levels of activity, and lose weight (if needed), they can significantly manage their diabetes. The treatment plan for type 2 may differ from person to person: one individual may need to take oral medication, another may not need to take medication and only needs to lose weight, and another may need to do both. The treatment plan will all depend on the medical and physical situation of that type 2 individual. A PWD with either type 1 or 2 diabetes will need to have a blood test every three months, known as the A1C. This test is to get a measure of the amount of sugar in the blood over the past two to three months. It's like a lie detector- the A1C results will tell the doctor how well this individual has been taking care of his or herself, or if the treatment plan is working. A good goal for a PWD is to have an A1C at 7% or lower.

For those with type 2 diabetes, there is even a possibility that a PWD who follows the doctor's treatment plan to perfection may be able to reduce or stop their medication completely; however, their high glucose numbers will return if they go back to their old, unhealthy habits. On the other hand, a diagnosis of type 1 diabetes means having this diagnosis for life, end of story. But keep on reading, there may not be a cure, but there is hope.

Chapter III: She Was My First

I did not get the news that I was pregnant that cold winter of 1991, but as the years have gone by and after becoming a parent of two boys, I associate living with T1D with parenting all the way. Imagine this: a young infant comes into your life and this infant remains an infant, dependent on you and only <u>YOU</u> forever. You must care for this infant with special needs forever and no one else can do this for you. Just you and only you!

<u>This is why I've declared that my diabetes was my first child.</u>

Let's talk about parenting and diabetes: Yes, pregnancy, having children, and parenting can all be beautiful things. These miracles occur every day and they are incredible experiences. Unlike becoming a parent, having diabetes is not a positive experience and I have struggled to find the miracle in it. Being told "you have diabetes" has none of the incredible feelings often associated with becoming a parent, such as excitement, joy, and love for this new phase in one's life.

So how is having diabetes like becoming a parent? The commonality that I see between having type 1 diabetes and becoming a parent is the fact that the disease is dependent on the person that has it. Even though the doctor did not give me the news of being pregnant in December 1991 or months later when I went from type 2 to type 1, I had to learn how to take care of my diabetes the same way I did when I had my handsome boys. This is why I call my diabetes my first child, my girl! Diabetes is something you'll have to care for; however, the big difference is that you <u>must do this forever</u>, otherwise the consequences will be horrific and devastating to one's health. When my diabetes turned 18 years old, it didn't go away to college. Living with T1D is like being the parent of an infant forever, an infant with very special needs who will never, ever grow up or mature.

Like having a dependent infant, having type 1 diabetes is always with you and will affect everything you do. Having T1D means that you wake up with diabetes, go to bed with diabetes, enter a relationship with diabetes, and when being intimate with your partner, *guess what*? Yes, diabetes will be right there with you. While you are sleeping, your diabetes is right there, but it is not sleeping. If you exercise, your diabetes is there as well. Regardless of what you do for a living and how you spend your time, your diabetes is right there, every step of the way and very active, I must say. No matter what you do, your diabetes will be there all the time, affecting you and requiring your time and attention. Unless a person with T1D gets a pancreas transplant, it will never, ever go away. If you are still wondering how type 1 diabetes is similar to caring for a child, continue to follow me in this journey.

Chapter IV: My Baby Bag

Just like with an infant, I can't ever leave home without packing a bag for my diabetes. I need a lot of things with me in order to properly care for my diabetes whenever it needs my attention, which is never predictable. First and most importantly, I need my glucometer with me at all times. A glucometer is a very smart and small device that tests and measures your blood glucose level when you give it a tiny, small drop of your blood. It's not a complicated device, anyone can use it once you learn the ins and outs of it. They come in all sizes, shapes, brands, and styles. It's critical to always use the same glucometer because it will store months of information for you, which can then be downloaded by you or by your doctor. From there, you can view your information in graphs, charts, and many other cool and helpful reports that you can discuss with your doctor.

Using this device is how I know if my blood glucose is high, within range, or low. This is how I know what I need to do and how I need to treat my diabetes. By using my glucometer often, I also get to learn how my body feels when I'm low, when I'm high, and when I'm okay. In my case, my glucometer is with me at all times. It's in my purse when I'm at work, in the car, at the boys' sports events, at church, at the stores, at the movies, I mean anywhere and everywhere. Most importantly, it is right next to my pillow when I sleep at night. I actually have more than one glucometer because if one breaks down, it's not something I can do without for a day or two. I also keep a spare one in my office in case I ever leave it at home, which has happened at least a handful of times in my T1D life of 30+ years.

Another very important item with me at all times is either a juice box or glucose tablets, which I use when my blood glucose becomes too low. Glucose tablets are just that: glucose/sugar, but it is fast-acting. They look like small candy, come in many different flavors, and are easy to store. They are inexpensive and convenient, you can buy them in bulk, and most importantly, they save lives. I like glucose tablets because they don't melt or freeze if you leave them in your car. I have a container of glucose tablets in my car and one in my husband's car. No matter where I am, I always have access to something that can raise my sugar whenever I may need it. You know that feeling you get when you are driving down your driveway and realize you don't have your cell phone with you? Well, something that can raise your sugar is just as important when you are living with T1D or T2D. At home and at work, I have juice boxes next to my bed and in my office. There are many other things that can raise your sugar, but the key thing is, it must be fast acting. I have used sugar envelopes (in desperate instances) and glucose gels in the past.

Think back to Chapter II: The Big Picture when you learned that a functioning pancreas produces both insulin and glucagon. Glucagon is a hormone that raises blood glucose levels. If you do not have diabetes and your pancreas detects that your glucose levels are low, your pancreas will know to release just the right amount of glucagon and communicate with your liver to release the stored glucose. This does not happen in someone that has type 1 diabetes. When I feel that my blood glucose is low, I need to take something to raise my blood glucose immediately. What I use to raise my blood glucose depends on where I am. For example, if I am at church, I would normally take glucose tablets (they are more discrete for this setting, but this does not mean, I could not drink a juice box). If I am working, I prefer to drink a juice box (I feel a juice box gets into my system much quicker and I don't need to chew anything). If it is in the middle of the night, I also go for the juice box; however, on rough nights (nights with too many lows), I may switch to glucose tablets because I don't want to keep waking up to go to the bathroom. ***The struggle is real!!***

Having a low is always an unpleasant experience (a whole chapter is dedicated to this topic and I will also discuss glucagon.) Having a low means that one's glucose level went from a normal level to a low level. What is a low glucose level? According to the Diabetes Association, a low glucose level is anything under 70mg[10]. Lows can range from mild to severe, even deadly. To me, every episode of low blood glucose is horrible. Lows are not good when waking up because it makes waking up much more difficult. Lows are not good in the middle of the day either; they interfere with anything you are trying to accomplish. Lows will interrupt anything you may be trying to focus and/or concentrate on. Lows will slow down your thoughts and suck your energy away. Lows are most definitely not good at nighttime when you are sleeping. Any low can be deadly, but having lows while you are sleeping can be not only dangerous, but terrifying. As you can see, there is never a good time to have a low. Lows are just as dangerous as highs but the difference is that you can feel the impact and consequences of a low right away. This is why a PWD, type 1 or 2, should always carry a form of glucose with them, to raise their blood glucose when experiencing a low.

The third thing I always carry with me is my form of treatment. In my case, my form of treatment is insulin, meaning that I have to use insulin to treat my diabetes, keeping my glucose levels within range. This is also known as being insulin-dependent. There are at least nine different types of insulin and which insulin I end up using as a form of treatment is decided by my doctor. In my years living with T1D, I have been on three different types of insulin.

The first 11.5 years of me living with T1D, I chose syringes to deliver my form of treatment (insulin). During these 11.5 years, I used two different types of insulin at different times of the day in order to treat my diabetes; therefore, during these years, I always had to carry my syringes and my insulin with me. If I was going to spend the night somewhere, I had to make sure I had my nighttime insulin with me, which was different from my daytime insulin. If I was going to be out in the sun, I had to make sure that my insulin was secured in a safe, cool container. Life was no longer a walk at the park or a day at the beach. I had to learn to do a lot of thinking and planning for my day, something I was NOT used to.

After 11.5 years, I grew tired of having to use syringes and I wanted to upgrade my insulin delivery system. I did some research, consulted with my healthcare team, and made up my mind to use a different delivery system: the insulin pump. The best way I can describe an insulin pump is to compare it to an intravenous device, like an IV line; however, the insulin is not being delivered to my veins, but to my bloodstream. To date, I have had two different types of insulin pumps. With my first insulin pump, I was attached to it almost constantly with a few exceptions: I had to remove it before showering, if I was going into a body of water, and before being intimate with my husband. With my current pump, however, I am literally attached to it 24 hours a day, 7 days a week. I can shower and go swimming with it, and I don't need to take it off during intimate moments. I remember going into surgery to have my 2nd C-Section and having to bring a letter from my diabetes team that informed my GYN doctors that it was okay for me to have my pump on during this procedure. My insulin pump is like my artificial pancreas.

Insulin pumps can seem very mysterious if you don't know anything about them. To me, the insulin pump has been liberating! My current insulin pump is wireless and has two pieces to it: the actual pump and a device that controls the pump. My wireless insulin pump fits on my palm. Once I fill it with insulin, I stick it on my body and then I use the other piece (I think of it as a remote) to tell it what the pump should do: how much insulin to give myself at specific hours and at meal times. After being on the pump for nine years, I decided to go back to basics, meaning I chose to go back to syringes. This did not last very long. I really enjoy the flexibility and freedom of having an insulin pump. One important thing to always remember is that this is *your* diabetes and you need to be involved and invested, researching your options in conjunction with your diabetes team.

Insulin pumps come in various styles and colors from different companies. They may have different features and functions, but they all do the same thing: deliver insulin into one's bloodstream. I feel blessed and privileged that I can benefit from such technology. The insulin pump is trying to do what a pancreas does and deliver insulin into my body 24/7. Based on my eating habits, exercise routine and lifestyle (active, sedentary, working, pregnant, hormonal, postmenopausal, whatever it may be,) my medical team and I came to an agreement on what **basal rate** my pump should deliver into my body. The basal rate is the rate of continuous insulin supply that the pump delivers into my body. Every time I see my medical team, this basal rate is reviewed and, if needed, it can be adjusted. In addition, I can have several basal rate programs stored in my insulin pump. For example, I can have a basal rate programmed for sick days, for PMS days, for weekends, and so on.

I can also tell the pump what **bolus** to give me. A bolus is the amount of insulin I tell the pump to give me when I am eating a meal and is also something my medical team and I determined together. The pump knows how much of a bolus to give me because it's been programmed to know the **insulin ratio** that is right for me for each meal. For example, I may have a ratio of 1:8 for breakfast. This means that for every 8 carbs in my meal, I need 1 unit of insulin to cover that. Depending on my body and the way it reacts to food at different times of the day and in different scenarios in my life, I may have different insulin ratios programmed in my pump. This is why it is critical for me to really know my diabetes and what different foods do to my body, and to thoroughly collect and document this data to share with my medical team so that we can determine the correct settings for my pump. Please keep in mind that even if one doesn't have an insulin pump or the desire to have one, it is still critical for one to really know their diabetes and what food does to their body, and to thoroughly collect and document this data to share with their medical team so they can determine the correct insulin ratio if they are type 1. It is also still critical for those with type 2 to fully understand their diabetes as this will help determine their treatment plan.

Besides my pump, I need to have everything that comes with the pump in case I need to change it or in case it runs out of insulin. This means I need to carry an extra pump set and an insulin bottle with me at all times. I always try to carry a couple of syringes with me just in case something goes really wrong with the pump. For my first pump, I also needed to have extra batteries at all times. For my current insulin pump, I need to charge it every night the way I charge my cell phone.

In addition, I have another amazing gadget called a continuous glucose monitor. A continuous glucose monitor is another device that gets topically inserted on my body and it measures my blood glucose level throughout the day and night. It has a separate piece called the receiver where I see my glucose number. The receiver fits on the palm of my hand. It can also be connected to my smartphone via an application. The information gathered by the receiver is information that I share with my medical provider. It is valuable information for my treatment. The continuous glucose monitor is wireless and I replace it every 10 days. I don't need to take it off to shower, to go into a body of water, or in intimate moments. There are various types of continuous glucose monitors, some can communicate with the insulin pump and some do not. I think of this device as lifesaving for me and is super essential in my treatment.

Lastly, there is one more thing I always have on me that can be very critical. This can also save your life if for some reason you find yourself unconscious and unable to speak for yourself. Regardless of what type of diabetes one has, a medical alert bracelet or necklace is essential to wear at all times. They now sell medical alert bracelets and necklaces of all kinds that are also quite lovely. Be sure to search for one that you would like to wear and invest in one.

So to make things easier for everyone, remember the most important things one needs, regardless of whether they are type 1 or 2, to manage one's diabetes can be as easy as 1, 2, 3, 4:

1. Glucometer

2. Glucose Tablets or any other form to treat a low

3. Form of treatment (insulin pump and/or syringes and insulin or pills)

4. A Medical Alert bracelet/necklace

The four tools above are critical tools one needs to manage one's diabetes, but the person with diabetes is the one in charge, they are the parent! When someone has a child, they become a parent. Well, when someone hears those words, "You have diabetes," they attain a new status as one living with diabetes and must always be prepared to properly care for it. They attain the status of becoming a Person With Diabetes.

Chapter V – Becoming a Person With Diabetes

Becoming a Type 1 PWD gave me a new responsibility to this new child of mine, who not only is with me, but lives *within me*. I need to keep up with medical appointments; yes, in the plural. In addition to my primary care doctor, I also see an endocrinologist (a diabetes specialist), a diabetes educator, a registered dietician, and an eye doctor. Depending on your health and if you have any other health complications, then your list of doctors could include additional specialists. For example, if you have a heart condition, then a cardiologist should be on your team of doctors. If you have problems with your kidneys, then an urologist needs to be part of your team.

Regardless of whether you wear eyeglasses, you should see an eye doctor at least once a year if you have diabetes. Why? Because diabetes affects your eyes. A foot doctor is another critical doctor to have on your team, regardless of if you are currently experiencing foot issues because diabetes can affect your feet. Both your podiatrist and endocrinologist will check your feet regularly. Why is this important? As I live with diabetes, I am aware that over time it can cause nerve damage (also known as diabetic neuropathy) and this can cause tingling sensations and pain in my feet. This can cause me to lose feeling in my feet. When this happens, if I step on something sharp like glass or a rock, or simply have a blister on my foot, I may not feel it. This can lead to cuts, sores, and infections, which over the years, if left untreated, can lead to other severe foot problems, such as amputations. Like I said before, diabetes affects you from head to toe!

Becoming a PWD (type 1 or 2) can make the PWD feel as if they are under a microscope with all of the doctors they must see. Needing all of these doctor's appointments is another way that caring for one's diabetes can be very similar to the care a responsible parent provides to their child. For example, it's recommended by The

American Academy of Pediatrics (AAP[11]) that babies get checkups at birth, then three to five days after birth and subsequently at one month, two months, four months, six months, nine months, twelve months, fifteen months, eighteen months, and twenty-four months of age. As babies get older, they most likely get seen once a year for a physical; with my diabetes, my doctor wants to see me at least twice a year, if not more.

There is one big difference between being a PWD and being a parent: I am not obligated to comply with my treatment plan and tend to my medical needs the way parents are required to care for their children. There isn't a child protective agency ensuring that I care for my diabetes, and no one can force me to comply with my doctor's recommendations. If I chose not to take care of my diabetes, my family and friends do not have a moral obligation to refer me to the doctor. Sadly, if I choose not to take care of my diabetes, I'm on my own and the consequences of such choices are life-threatening and serious.

It is up to the PWD to choose to engage in their treatment and do what is needed and recommended. An endocrinologist can tell his/her patient everything that has to be done, prescribe the right medicines and tools, and provide the proper services and staff, but a PWD may continue to struggle with their diabetes and have difficulty engaging in more productive self-management behaviors. I must say that I am not perfect when it comes to my diabetes. In all honesty, taking care of my diabetes has proven to be very challenging, overwhelming, stressful, exhausting, and very frustrating. But every day, I aim to make healthy choices. Some days I get close to that goal, some days I don't. But that is my *daily* goal.

If I want my diabetes, or my child as I refer to it, to be successful, not only should I follow the expert's advice, but I also need to realize that I, the person with T1D, have the biggest role in this story. I am in charge of my diabetes. If you are a PWD, you know every day is never, ever the same. One of the biggest reasons why I need to be in charge is the fact that I know myself better than anyone else. I know what works and what doesn't work for me.

I refer to my diabetes as my daughter with "special needs." My diabetes needs my constant attention and care. She will never mature, nor leave me or my home. She will be with me 24/7 until my death. Another great disadvantage of my diabetes is that no one can help me care for her. I cannot drop her off at the sitter for a few hours, nor can I bring her to daycare while I go to work. If I go on vacation, there are no grandmas or aunts and uncles or big sisters that can take care of her while I go on a second honeymoon. I cannot leave her with my husband while I go shopping or out with the girls. *I AM THE SOLE HUMAN BEING WHO CAN TAKE CARE OF HER.*

Unfortunately, my diabetes, my first child, does not mature or grow up the way most children do. In my case, my stepchildren are now adults and successfully independent. My 22-year-old son is in graduate school and my 17-year-old son is starting his freshman year in college. Unlike my diabetes, my children have advanced in life, constantly growing and maturing, and becoming very independent. My diabetes will never, ever get to that level. As a matter of fact, I find that the older I get, the more difficult my diabetes becomes. The older I get, the less tolerant my body becomes of certain foods. The older I get, the harder it gets for me to manage my diabetes; however, as I do for my own children, one thing I can do for my diabetes is HOPE for her to be successful in life. After all, her success will truly reflect on me and on my health. Of course, I have to adjust my expectations for her. My diabetes will never get an education. My diabetes is not capable of learning anything, so I'm not able to educate her on how she should behave, like I've done with our children. This means my diabetes can be challenging but I can learn. I can train myself to eat differently, to live differently, and to make better choices.

If looking at diabetes as a child is not something you can relate to, then look at it as your career goals, your aspirations in life. If I want my diabetes to be successful, I need to set some goals for her. Just like with setting career goals, I need to focus on and work towards achieving my diabetes goals. The same way you collaborate with your co workers or get support and supervision from your boss, you will collaborate with and get support and supervision from your medical team.

As in everything in life, nothing comes easy. Caring for one's diabetes is hard work. Not only is it hard work, it is constant, everlasting, never-ending work that must be assessed and evaluated, and goals and expectations will need to be adjusted. Just like when I went to college with the plan to be a medical doctor only to change my mind after taking a chemistry class, there has to be room for change when it comes to diabetes. With careers and life, there has to be room for the unexpected, room for that accident or illness no one saw coming. With diabetes, there has to be room for the time you forgot to take that insulin shot with your meal or you miscalculated the carbs in your meal, or better yet, regardless of the nutritional facts label, your body said otherwise and ended up with a 300 glucose number. As a PWD, one has to be willing to make changes on a regular basis, like one may change departments in their company or actually change careers. One has to be willing to go with the punches, every second.

In a nutshell, a PWD needs to be flexible, among many other things because diabetes brings a whole new aspect to your life. I like to refer to it as one needing to have mental flexibility. It doesn't really matter how old the PWD is, diabetes will change their life forever. In my case, in my most humble moments, I can honestly say that my diabetes saved me from living a very unhealthy lifestyle.

For now, let's focus on setting goals. For my diabetes, my first child, my daughter, these are my goals for her:

- Attain and maintain an A1C no higher than 6.5 (I've learned that the older I get, the harder this goal becomes.)

- Maintain a good cholesterol level, one that will keep me from developing heart disease.

- Continue to have the ability to handle my own treatment
  o As I age, I want to be able to navigate carb counting and the technology available for diabetes treatment. I can only dream of what the technology for diabetes will look like in 30 years when I'll be 82!

- Continue to exercise!
  o Believe it or not, exercise can be a natural medicine for PWDs, but not every form of

exercise has the same effect. Again, each individual is different and only the individual can learn how exercise benefits him/her. My goal is to be active for life.

- Continue making changes in my eating habits and maintain these changes, which will lead me to attain and maintain a healthy weight.

- Decrease my chances of developing other health complications due to my diabetes, such as but not limited to: depression, high blood pressure, becoming overweight, blindness, heart disease, amputations, kidney failure, and many, many other sad complications[12].

The goals I want to attain can be very challenging and hard to achieve; however, I find the following key factors to be very important and critical to my success:

- Stay positive

- Stay physically active

- Be your best advocate: do your own research and ask questions at your follow-up appointments, ask why and how things work.

- Find support: diabetes is 100% overwhelming for the PWD. Don't hesitate to look for professional mental health support if you are feeling like you are overwhelmed with the demands of your diabetes.

- Work with your medical team

- Don't ever give up!

In retrospect, on that cold, dreary day in December of 1991, life could have dealt me worse cards than my diagnosis as a person with diabetes. But at that time in my life, I was still young and not wise enough to realize such a thing. It did take me a long time to make the permanent changes that my body needed me to make. It also seemed like a very long time before I found the right endocrinologist. I remember that search like it was yesterday. It was almost like dating and looking for the right partner!

Chapter VI: Finding Mr. or Mrs. Right

Now, as you may recall, I went to a walk-in clinic and was diagnosed with type two diabetes. There was no endocrinologist at the clinic; therefore, I was advised to get one. What is an endocrinologist? An endocrinologist is a medical expert who specializes in treating diabetes and other diseases of the endocrine system. Our pancreas, a very critical organ in our bodies, is part of the endocrine system. In the case of someone like me, my pancreas stopped producing insulin, thus making me a person with T1D. Although the endocrinologist is the medical expert, I have learned this does not mean you have no say in your treatment. Ultimately, if you manage your diabetes and work cooperatively with a medical team, you will become the expert of your own diabetes because you are the one who lives with the diabetes 24/7.

Finding an endocrinologist I felt comfortable with was a challenging experience. To me, it was worse than dating! I wanted the perfect match for me; however, this proved to be no easy task. The first endocrinologist I met was from a list provided to me by my insurance. I don't remember his name, but I can still picture his office in my mind. It was a cold environment, very rigid-looking and unwelcoming. I vaguely remember what he looked like and very clearly remember that I did not like the things this doctor said to me. The point of the matter was not whether he was correct at the time, it was what he said, how he said it, and how he addressed me.

During my first visit, this doctor told me I had to stop eating meat or I would end up having to use INSULIN. Remember, at this time I had not been properly diagnosed. That was a very scary word for me to hear back then. Almost 99.9% of the time when I met someone and they learned I had been diagnosed with type 2 diabetes, he or she would give me the following response: *"Oh...well, at least you don't have the bad one, the one with the needles."* I was terrified of having to go on insulin and I definitely didn't want to give up eating meat. At that time in my life, I was known to be a huge meat-eater. You could've called me Marie the T-Rex. The thought of having to give up meat AND using insulin was terrifying to me. It was bad enough I had just been diagnosed with diabetes, had to give up sugar and candy, take pills, and poke my fingers for blood daily, and now he wanted me to give up meat? Was he crazy? He sure did not have any compassion for me and if he did, he showed it the wrong way. I didn't see it, I didn't feel it.

The ironic thing is that, 14 years later, I decided to give up meat. I made this decision on my own, at my own time, based on my own research. It was my choice. Just like a therapist begins to work with his/her client where the client is at that time, this endocrinologist should have done the same. He should've begun working with me where I was at that time. In retrospect, I was lost back then. I was overwhelmed, scared, and confused, and he should have started working with me on the very basics. He moved along too fast for me at that time. I think I only went to that doctor once or twice. Then, a blessing in disguise took place: my employer made some changes in health insurance and I was forced to pick a different medical insurance. With this change, I also had to see a different doctor. Thank GOD, I thought to myself.

While my medical insurance was changing, another change was taking place in my body: I began to lose a lot more weight and once again, I was not feeling good. I was tired and this time, I even missed my menstrual period, which was not like me at all. I began the dating game and searched for a new doctor through my new insurance.

This time, I found myself in a wonderful setting. I can remember it as if it was yesterday. It was one facility with a lot of different doctors. *It was heavenly.* My new primary doctor ran some tests, then told me the most terrible news I could have heard at that time in my life: my blood work was out of control and I could have died. Bottom line, I needed to go on insulin immediately. My type 2 diabetes was now type 1. Just like that, I was not given any time to think about it. There I was, not pregnant and facing my worst nightmare becoming a reality.

Thankfully, my new primary doctor made it possible for me to get an appointment with the most wonderful human being I would meet at this time in my life: my first diabetes educator. I can honestly say as time went by, she became a very good friend and I was blessed to have her in my life. Along with my brand new and first ever diabetes educator, I also met my new endocrinologist. This was the beginning of my life with T1D and, most importantly, I had a team on my side. I had a primary doctor, an endocrinologist, and a diabetes educator, all in the same building. They were like my second family and believe it or not, every single one of them truly cared about my health and my well-being. This team was key to my success.

If I had to give you any advice regarding your search for an endocrinologist, I would say do your research. Remember, it is *your* diabetes and health. Your success with your diabetes will depend not only on you, but also on the team of doctors that are working with you; this is critical for any PWD. Also, keep in mind that it is either your insurance or your out-of-pocket money paying for their services, so why not put some effort into finding the right doctor? I was too young back then to realize this and I just accepted things as they fell into my lap. I must have had an angel looking out for me because I ended up in good hands and it was a huge blessing for me and my diabetes. Remember that it is important for you to advocate for yourself!

Chapter VII: The First Date

My first appointment with my new diabetes educator was a wonderful experience for me. I remember my first appointment like it was yesterday. I remember what the office looked like, it was warm and inviting. Most of all, I remember that we began to talk and she asked me a lot of questions so she could get to know me. As this process was taking place, I realized my fears were beginning to decrease. This was it! The first sign that I was experiencing a match made in heaven.

This wonderful human being wanted to know me as a person. She wanted to know what changes I had made for myself in the past year. My new diabetes educator did not have an abrasive style, and was clear, honest, kind, and firm in the sweetest possible way. This wonderful human being made the transition from type 2 to type 1 so easy that it made me feel strong; it made me feel confident that I could truly do this. One of the most valuable lessons she taught me was how to identify and treat an episode of low blood glucose levels. I still remember my first low; sadly, it happened before I met my first diabetes educator. The saddest and scariest thing was that I had no clue what I was experiencing. I was at the gym (trying to stay fit) on the treadmill and I suddenly felt "weird." That was the only way I could describe it at the time. I felt like my eyes couldn't see straight, my heart was beating a little faster. Unfortunately for me, I had not met my first diabetes educator yet and I had not been educated on how to recognize a low.

My purse and glucometer were in the car so I went to the car, checked my blood glucose levels and bingo, I was low. What do I do now? I asked myself. I did not have any glucose tablets with me, I didn't even know what glucose tablets were back then. I didn't have any juice or candy either, and I didn't have any cash on me. Suddenly my heart starts beating a little faster, now I'm afraid. Luckily for me, I found some loose change in my car and I was able to go back to the gym and get an apple-cranberry juice. It was a very frightening experience, one I could've been better equipped to handle had I been properly educated. From that day on, my gym bag not only carried my glucometer, but also some change and something to raise my sugar.

My diabetes educator taught me that I have to carry my glucometer with me at ALL TIMES. I was also taught that the days of having a tiny purse were OVER because I needed to be prepared to care for my diabetes. Again, as the years went on, this is how I came to the conclusion that my diabetes was my first child. I always have to be prepared to care for this child at any time of the day and anywhere I find myself. That means that my glucometer, my insulin, my glucose tablets, and much more need to be in that "baby bag" A.K.A. my purse. I must admit that, despite all the new stuff I was learning from my diabetes educator, it took a few years for me to actually get into a routine and to seriously be prepared for my diabetes at all times.

My diabetes educator also taught me how to inject myself in the least painful ways. I was introduced to a device that made injecting myself easier (yes, that was possible). I would put the syringe with the insulin needed inside of this device. What made it easier was the fact that I really did not get to see much of the needle as it was going into my body. If you are a PWD, it's important that the people you live with also know how to inject you in case they ever need to, especially the glucagon (I will talk more about this life-saving device in a later chapter.) As the years went by and I began to take my diabetes care more seriously, my diabetes educator stressed the importance of those living with me also being educated on diabetes. One great suggestion I was given was to attend a class with a dietician. Although my now-husband and I were only dating at that time, we both agreed it was important for him to come along to the class with the dietician and my diabetes educator. We both learned a lot. For the first time in my life, I learned to measure food.

My new diabetes educator suggested that I carry some measuring cups in my purse until I got used to food measurements, and I did for a while. Believe me, half a cup is not that much at all. It's amazing how much food we are accustomed to eating while being clueless about the actual amount of food, calories, and carbohydrates we are consuming. For the first time in my life, I saw food as fuel to my body and not so much as satisfaction to every craving. It took many, many years before I accepted the fact that it is best to view food only as fuel, and my biggest struggle to this day is to not view food as comfort!

Chapter VIII: Diabetes and Its Hidden Demons: The Low Demon

Even though I consider my diabetes my first child, I'm not in love with her the way I fell in love with my boys when I first laid eyes on them when they were born. I can honestly say that I dislike my diabetes and I often feel my diabetes is possessed. Yes, you read that correctly: my diabetes is possessed! I can never predict her behavior and when she misbehaves, I don't ever think it is cute or funny and it is NEVER, EVER GOOD! To me, one of the hidden demons in diabetes is the Demon of Low Glucose Numbers, also known as hypoglycemia.

Like I said before, there is never a good time to have a low. The consequences of a low are felt immediately. A low blood glucose level will have many different personalities and none of them are pretty. As time goes by, they take different shapes, forms, and personalities, presenting in many, many different ways. I've noticed that the older I get, the harder it is for me to recognize a low. This is why it is critical that one checks their blood glucose often, day and night. This way, one becomes familiar with the many personalities of a low.

The personalities of a low will be different for everyone. For me, the first thing that goes when I'm having a low is the brain, meaning my ability to think straight. I feel disoriented, confused, and unable to perform simple tasks. A simple question like, "What day of the week is it today?" can be difficult to answer. My answer will most likely be, "Wait, I can't think of it right now" or "Not now, honey," but the sweet tone may be absent. The only thing that the brain can focus on during a low is, "What can I eat? I have to eat NOW!" The scary thing is that even when that personality appears, you can still not realize that you are having a low.

I recall a particular episode that occurred while grocery shopping with my husband. We were at the checkout line putting our groceries onto the belt. Suddenly, I felt this desperate urge to eat a bag of peanut M&M's.

Of course, it did not help to see all the candies at the register. I grabbed a bag and started gobbling down the M&M's as I threw our items into the belt. My husband looked at me and asked if I was okay. I answered him kind of brusquely, "Yeah, why?" He replied, "Well, you're kind of killing that whole bag of M&M's like it's your last meal." A light bulb went off and I checked my blood sugar when we got to the car. Bingo, it was low. And in case you were wondering, I paid for the M&M's.

Another way a low can show itself is in one's behavior. During a low, it's like one has lost the ability to tolerate anything. Your behavior can be very quick-tempered, irritable, and impatient. The way I've interpreted this over the years is that my body is demanding my attention because it wants something right away, but it doesn't know how to communicate this to me (much like a child.) This is my body saying, "Please, feed me something sweet because

I'm low and do it NOW." I have heard of people who have found out about their diabetes when they have observed a strange shift in their behavior and chose to seek medical advice.

Another way in which a low can present itself is in one's energy level. You can be fine at one point and then feel completely depleted of energy ten minutes later. I remember being at a wedding with my husband once. We were inside the church and I had left everything in the car: my purse, glucometer, glucose tablets, and insulin. In a nutshell, everything I knew I should always carry with me. But I was at a wedding and when your purse looks like a baby bag, it's not the prettiest accessory to bring along. Anyway, my husband suddenly looked at me and asked if I was okay. He said that my body was sinking into the pew, my shoulders were just fading away, and I seemed drained. I wondered what my sugar level was so I went out to the car (you'd think by now I would've learned my lesson that you never, EVER leave your glucometer behind.) I checked my glucose and there it was, I was low, somewhere in the 50's. I consumed some glucose tablets and within 15 minutes, I was a new woman. How many glucose tablets to consume when having a low is a conversation for you and your endocrinologist to have.

Something that can impact how a low presents itself is the time of day. For example, if my low is happening during the time I'm about to wake up, guess what? I may not want to get out of bed. I may be overly sleepy or sluggish, feel extremely tired or physically weak. At this point in my diabetes (30 years), I know that this is most likely a low, so I make an effort to wake up, reach for my continuous glucose monitor, and confirm that I am low. But believe me that this effort does not happen easily. I could lay there for minutes, telling myself how tired I am, how I need more sleep. At times, I may not even hear the beeping of my continuous glucose monitor. Before I had my continuous glucose monitor, if I was experiencing a low during my waking hours, I would just keep snoozing the alarm on my cell phone because, like I said before, the ability to think straight goes right out the window. I used to tell my husband, "If you see me turning the alarm off over and over again when both of us know I should be up because I have places to be, please tell me to check my sugar." I've also experienced waking up in a low after dreaming that I was eating and eating, unable to satisfy an intense hunger.

One other way to describe how a low can present itself in a PWD is when one experiences a food binge. I believe this personality is a combination of many other personalities and is more like a monster. During a low, you experience a very desperate need to eat something immediately, feeling like you'll die if you don't eat right then. Unfortunately, what usually happens on these occasions is that one tends to overeat because it takes a while for that desperate, awful, scary, and overwhelming feeling to go away. The consequence of going on this eating binge is that you will end up having to fix a high hours later because you overdid it! Once again, the ability to think straight is the first thing to go out the window and all those scary feelings literally take you over.

As you can see, there can be several personalities of a low; however, there are two I fear the most. The first one is the low that shows up in the middle of the night while I'm in my deepest stage of sleep. If I don't wake up from this low, I can go into a coma or even die. To this day, I have been blessed to always wake up from a low but I guarantee you, it is never a pretty sight. During the early years of me living with diabetes, I used to wake up sweating, shaking, frantic, and confused. I also remember the first time I lived in an apartment that had a garbage disposal. Believe it or not, I had never had a garbage disposal before then and don't ask me why, but I was intimidated by it. I did not like the power it had to demolish food. So, for a very long time, whenever

I would wake up to a low, I thought the sound of the garbage disposal was what woke me up. I would wake up sweaty with my heart racing, sit straight up in my bed and quickly realize that I was not hearing the garbage disposal and was actually experiencing a low. That is what I call divine intervention! I am at a point in my diabetes where I no longer experience lows like this. These lows show up without the sweating, shaking, heart palpitations, and confusing feelings. This is called hypoglycemia unawareness[13]. In the past, my dogs have woken me up and may GOD bless them for that. Besides the dogs, I now also have technology that helps with these lows (more to come on technology in a later chapter.)

The second low that I fear the most is the low that can show up while I'm driving. I categorize these two lows as *almost* equally dangerous and scary because I happen to be very vulnerable during these times. I say "almost" because the driving low is the scariest one to me.

I may have my family with me or I can hurt someone else. The terrifying thing is that these lows can creep up so quietly and so suddenly. While driving, you may suddenly find yourself disoriented, you might develop a headache, your vision may get blurry, and you may be unable to focus on the road. Once again, your brain's ability seems to be diminished. Before the technology that I have today, I would make it a point to check my glucose before I began to drive. If you don't have a continuous glucose monitor, I would say it is very important to always check your blood glucose before driving a vehicle. If you start to feel "weird" (dizzy, extremely tired, blurred vision, suddenly hot and sweaty) while driving, please find a way to safely pull your car over in a safe location and check your glucose.

Lows can disguise themselves in so many ways. No one tells you about these various personalities and perhaps the reason for this is that if you are not a PWD, you don't really know the ins and outs of diabetes.

Even medical experts cannot warn you as to which personalities you will experience because the ways in which lows are experienced varies from PWD to PWD. One thing that I have learned is that everything I do will affect my diabetes. Even sex will affect your diabetes. Sex can often be a workout and during a workout, you sweat and burn energy, which means a PWD's glucose levels go down.

It is very important that one understands that lows can happen anytime, anywhere and they can be very unpredictable. The lesson to be learned in this chapter is that every PWD will experience diabetes in their very own unique way, which is why anyone with diabetes should constantly check their blood glucose so they can learn the personalities of their lows. This is the only way one gets to know one's diabetes, one's body, and how one reacts to different foods and different activities. Also, please remember that diabetes ages with us and as we age, our bodies change.

Women in particular have a great deal of hormonal changes as they age and these changes impact one's diabetes. As this aging process occurs, the demands and personalities of our diabetes also change. So, just because you know that one cup of rice requires x-amount of insulin today, this may not always be the case.

You may be wondering how often lows happen. This will also vary from PWD to PWD. For me, I have multiple lows every week; however, I work really hard to avoid lows in the middle of the night because that's when I'm more vulnerable. How do I accomplish this? I don't experiment with foods I've never had at dinner or in the evenings. During these times, I also stay away from foods I know will cause a rollercoaster of ups and downs.

I can't stress enough how important it is to constantly check your blood glucose levels. My current pump does not recognize I am having a low, only the continuous glucose monitor recognizes this. The pump will continue to give me my background insulin unless I tell it to stop giving me insulin. If I want to give myself insulin while I am having a low **and** I tell the pump I am having a low, then the pump will give me a message that it cannot calculate a bolus for me because my blood glucose is either too low or too high. As you can see, it is critical to check one's blood glucose as often as possible. After living with diabetes for over 30 years, I've come to realize that lows have many different personalities so anytime I suspect I may be experiencing a low, I always:

1. Check my glucose (however, if you feel so low that you are about to faint, immediately treat the low)

2. Confirm a low

3. Treat a low

The above order is critical!

Chapter IX: Diabetes and Its Other Hidden Demon:

The High Demon

As I said in the previous chapter, I often feel as if my diabetes is possessed and has many personalities. Another terrifying hidden demon that I've experienced over the past 30 years is the Demon of the High Glucose Numbers, also known as hyperglycemia. Having high numbers is also a deadly matter and it has many horrific consequences; however, unlike the low demon, the consequences of high glucose numbers are not always seen immediately. This is how diabetes, when not well-managed, will slowly kill the human body.

Like the lows, the Demon of the Highs also has many personalities and these manifest in a variety of ways. By nature, I'm a cheery, energetic, positive, and happy-go-lucky kind of person; therefore, the one manifestation of the high demon I despise the most are the times when my mood turns depressive, gloomy, sad, impatient, short tempered, and/or easily annoyed. Each time I felt this way before having the technology that I have today, I would run for my glucometer because, again, by nature, that's just not me. Once I checked my blood glucose, sure enough I happened to be high. This is the one personality of the high demon that I could do without. It truly changes me and affects me in a negative way. It puts me in a miserable mood. With my fingertips as witnesses since I constantly check my glucose, I often recognize these changes in me.

Another high manifestation is in my energy levels. I've experienced being high in the 250+ range and when this has occurred, I have felt extremely drained and exhausted, like a sleepy cloud had fallen over me. Keep in mind that blood glucose levels within a healthy range for a PWD are 80-130 before a meal and less than 180 two hours after the start of a meal.[14] Again, I would have not learned to identify these symptoms if I was not constantly checking my blood glucose. I hope I'm clearly sending the message of how critical it is for a PWD to constantly check his/her blood glucose, particularly if you don't have the technology of a continuous glucose monitor.

High glucose numbers can manifest in many different ways. Just like a low, it all depends on the time of the day and what one may be doing. Again, the only way you will know yourself, how your body feels during these episodes, is if you are constantly observing and monitoring your glucose, especially when things feel off. For example, another way the high demon can make itself known is when I get crazy cravings without that "desperate to eat" feeling I described earlier. For some odd reason, I crave foods I know I should not eat during a high: candy, sweets, potato chips, and chocolate, and it's not due to me being on my menses. When this feeling arises, I check my blood glucose and find that I'm high. To this day, I still do not understand this manifestation! I can see how such a manifestation would make sense if I was having a low, but it does NOT make any sense for these symptoms to present when my blood glucose is high.

I have experienced other symptoms such as headaches, extreme thirst, frequent visits to the bathroom, bad breath, and a bad taste in my mouth, and there may be other symptoms I have yet to experience. There is one very important symptom I want to discuss in depth: depression. I am a therapist and depression is something I unfortunately deal with on a daily basis with different clients. When I was first diagnosed with diabetes, I did a lot of research and one thing that quickly alarmed me was the studies that linked diabetes to depression and found that people with diabetes are at risk of becoming depressed. Having a family history of depression and other mental health issues made these findings much more alarming. I can attest that when my glucose is high, I feel sad, helpless, and sometimes very depressed. These feelings are very powerful and I often struggle to make sense of them. The next paragraph is my attempt to make sense of them.

I am sure you would agree that food brings a great deal of emotional comfort. As a PWD, I have a very conflicted relationship with food; eating is no longer simple. This reality by itself is frustrating. I feel sad and blue when I am surrounded by delicious foods and I in good consciousness cannot eat any of it. I often think, "I want to eat food without consequences," but that is not my reality. It is very depressing when I venture past my safest meal (salad with a fish), work diligently in carb counting, and give myself the "right" amount of insulin, only to end up with a high glucose number three hours later. It is depressing when I eat a familiar "safe" dish and treat it with the usual amount of insulin and this one time, I end up high because God only knows why. It is very frustrating when I realize my glucose is high because I got distracted with life and I didn't take insulin with my meal. I have had many moments when I have been so frustrated, so annoyed and upset with my high numbers that I've made statements such as, "I'm done with this," "I give up," "I hate my life," and worse.

My most depressing moment was when I went to the eye doctor and after 30 years of living with T1D, my eye doctor told me that I have mild nonproliferative retinopathy.[15] This is the first stage of PWD eye disease. This means that I have small bulges in the small blood vessels of my retinas. These bulges are known as microaneurysms and they can cause the vessels to leak small amounts of blood into my retinas. This hit me hard because, in my opinion, I work very hard to be healthy. Of course, I am not perfect but I have made some serious changes in my diet and in my lifestyle. I felt judged when the doctor said, "You need to control your diabetes to avoid these spots from getting worse." I didn't respond, I was in shock. In my head, I was saying, "What do you think I do every day? You try living in my shoes for 30 days." I was angry, then sad, then depressed. My paternal grandmother (Mamá, may her soul rest in peace) became blind at the age of 25. It is not clear what caused her blindness since it happened a long time ago (she was born in 1903 and lived to the age of 106,) but I do know she was not a PWD. With having blindness in my family, this new diagnosis of mild nonproliferative retinopathy hit my heart and soul very sharply, and it really shook me to my core. I went to a retina specialist at the suggestion of my first diabetes educator (now a very good friend) and this doctor did not see anything different. I felt relieved that the diagnosis was not worse, but was still devastated and disappointed. As for the eye doctor, I didn't go back to her. In my opinion, she was not sympathetic and just assumed that I hadn't been taking care of my diabetes. Thankfully, this particular practice is large and I was able to choose a more sympathetic eye doctor.

I feel blessed that I can bring myself back to the other side of these depressive thought patterns and I can start all over; not everyone can do that. How do I manage my frustrating moments, my dark moments? I have a supportive family. I surround myself with people who want to be healthy. I meditate and do yoga to keep my stress levels somewhat manageable. I aim to live a purposeful life and I am always working to improve myself. I have a strong faith in God and I pray for creativity and energy. Because I am a therapist, I do have other therapists that I can talk to, bounce things off of to help maintain my sanity. It's work and it's daily work!

If you are a PWD and you are feeling depressed, extremely overwhelmed, anxious, and sad too often, please seek the professional help of a mental health therapist. Not only would it be good for your diabetes to get things on track, but it would make you feel great all around. High glucose numbers can make you feel depressed, but just having diabetes can make you feel very depressed. The disease of diabetes is very overwhelming and it affects your health from head to toe, inside and outside. The lifestyle changes you are expected to make are huge, but critical. Don't forget about the damage that consistent high numbers can do to your overall health.

Chapter X: Dealing with Highs and Lows in the Diabetes Rollercoaster

You know, there are times that I tell myself, "Diabetes is not so bad. It's not cancer, it's not Alzheimer's, it's not MS. It's not like I immediately lost my limbs, my eyesight, or the ability to speak. I'm just living with diabetes. Being a PWD in this era, in this century, sure is much better than it was 100 years ago. After all, I don't have to boil glass needles, I don't have to urinate on a stick. I can live. I can do this." And yes, I'm partially right: caring for diabetes can be done, but it requires a lot of work, commitment, and discipline from the individual affected by it. Please remember that the most evil thing about diabetes is that it will slowly kill you if you do not follow your treatment and get a handle on it. It will destroy your body slowly and you will suffer along the way. Diabetes, the possessed disease as I also like to call it, is a powerful disease. It does not ever go into remission and, to date, does not have a cure. Diabetes, most definitely, has many personalities of its own.

Both high and low blood glucose numbers are very dangerous and it's important to prevent them and to be prepared to manage them if/when they occur. The hidden demons of diabetes, the high and low demons, can be somewhat tamed. Just like a child, diabetes needs discipline, structure, and consistency. These components are critical when one has diabetes and should always be present in any treatment for one's diabetes, whether the treatment is followed via insulin, diet, or medication. As a T1D, my doctor and I have agreed on an **insulin-to-carbohydrate ratio**. This means that I will take 1 unit of insulin for a certain amount of carbohydrates (carbs). I have tools with me that tell me how many carbohydrates are in various foods; however, there are times when I don't know exactly how many carbs are in a meal. When this happens, I'm the one deciding how much insulin my body needs for that meal or for that snack. When I do this critical role on my own, I may not always be that precise and I may end up with a low or high blood glucose.

Let's start by discussing the lows. There are multiple factors that can cause a low. For example, I can go low because I worked out a bit harder than usual, or the temperature was hotter than usual that day, thus my body was working harder. My pancreas is not able to give me the glucagon I need. The bottom line is that a PWD, particularly those with T1D, will inevitably experience a low at some point. Each low has its level of severity and this all depends on a couple of key aspects:

1. The speed of the low as it's happening. If I go from a glucose level of 130 to 100 in 20 minutes, I will physically feel that low, and heavily. I may experience sweaty hands, a racing heart, and other physical symptoms. To drop 30 points in 20 minutes is very significant.

2.   The timing of the low. My response to a low will be different if I experience a drop of 30 points in 20 minutes while I am awake at the office compared to when I am in the deepest sleep stage.

I have a funny story to share with you (well, it is funny now). Ten years into my diabetes, I went on a family trip to Puerto Rico. The weather was much warmer than it was at home (factor # 1). We were out of our routine and were eating different foods, being more physically active, and not keeping my usual eating schedule and diet (big factor # 2). I was also under a lot of stress and was mentally and physically exhausted (factor # 3). We were staying at my parents' home and my husband, my two year old, and I were sharing a bed. I woke up in the middle of the night, mumbling something to my husband as I tried to sit up in bed, but there wasn't much room. I finally got out of bed literally half asleep, walked to my son's baby bag in the living room, and took out what I thought was my bottle of glucose tablets. At this time in my life, I literally used my son's baby bag as my diabetes baby bag. It was my way of simplifying my life. I went back to the bedroom and tried to open the glucose bottle but I couldn't open it. My husband saw me struggling and quickly realized that I didn't have the bottle of glucose tablets in my hand; I had a plastic toy horse that belonged to my son.

Later, I found out that my husband started panicking because he thought I was losing my mind. He realized what was happening when I explained that my glucose tablets wouldn't open and got me a glass of orange juice. Somehow, in the midst of all of this, I managed to check my blood glucose and my husband and I saw that I had a 55 glucose level. A few minutes after drinking the orange juice, I was back to being myself and we laughed at that scary moment. I might've had a speedy low, but the most critical factor here was the *timing* of this low. I was probably in some serious deep sleep and thus unable to quickly realize I was having a low that needed to be treated. I also did not have the technology I have today. Had this same low happened during the day, I would've been able to handle it in a much better and safer manner.

Now let's discuss the highs. The severity of a high depends on how consistently I get to a high range. As a reminder, anything above 180 is considered high; however, the timing of a 180+ glucose reading matters. If I have a 180 glucose reading two hours after the start of a meal versus a 180 glucose reading when I wake up in the morning, these are two totally different scenarios. The 180 glucose reading as I am fasting is a dangerous reading compared to the 180 glucose reading two hours after I started a meal. There are appropriate glucose ranges for when one is fasting, and for 2 hours after a meal and before meals. According to the Diabetes Association, a PWD should ideally maintain "tight control" on their glucose levels and keep them between 70 and 130 mg/dl before meals, and less than 180 mg/dl two hours after one has started a meal. "Tight control" means aiming to get numbers as close to what a person without diabetes would have.[16] Having a 180 glucose reading two hours after a meal makes sense because my body is still processing the meal, whereas I would be concerned about what was causing a fasting 180 glucose reading.

I follow the same process when it comes to dealing with both lows and highs, though the actual treatment will differ:

1. Always be prepared- I always have my tools and baby bag within reach.

2. Check my blood glucose at crucial times and as soon as I start to suspect I may be low or high.

3. Have a form of treatment handy

My glucometer, insulin pump, and continuous glucose monitor are with me at all times, whether I'm at home, work, or out and about. As discussed in an earlier chapter, I can't ever leave home without my diabetes baby bag because I always need to monitor and be prepared to manage my diabetes. I may sound like a broken record but I cannot stop emphasizing how vital it is for a PWD to constantly check their blood glucose. The more you know yourself, the greater your chances will be of recognizing when you may be low or high. Before I had all the technology I have today, I would check my blood glucose often and at crucial times. I still do, just not as often.

Crucial times are immediately upon waking, when fasting, before each meal, two hours after each meal, before bedtime, and ideally in the middle of the night. Why these times? These times are significant because this is how I learn if I am using the right amount of insulin. This is also how I learn what foods I am more sensitive to. Before I was introduced to all the technology I have today (more on this in a later chapter,) my rule was, if I open my mouth to eat anything, I check my blood glucose before I eat. I also sleep with my glucometer, insulin pump, and continuous glucose monitor right under my pillow or next to my pillow. Because 99.9% of the time when I wake up with a low, I'm tired, sluggish, and disoriented, I sometimes leave my meter ready with a clean strip. This helps me avoid looking for and inserting a test strip in the dark. The more you know yourself and the more you understand your body and your diabetes' many personalities, the better your chances will be of preventing your blood glucose from being high or drastically low.

I also check my glucose before and after any physical activity, including sex. Checking my glucose at these times is very critical and helps me avoid lows and keep my glucose within range. Believe it or not, exercise is like a natural medicine for a PWD. Sex can and almost always will lower your blood glucose, it's a workout! While exercise will lower your blood glucose level, how long its effect lasts depends on the type of exercise you do. For example, my glucose levels react differently to aerobics versus strength training. Because I have been experimenting with this aspect of my life for some time now (I experimented by checking my glucose levels before, during, and after exercise,) I know how my body reacts to different types of exercises. I've also come to learn when not to use insulin, when to decrease the amount of insulin, and when to make changes to my basal rates in my insulin pump. My basal rate can be different throughout the day. For example, my basal rate is different while I'm sleeping versus during the day when I'm awake. With the technology in my pump, I am able to adjust my basal rate as needed. If I didn't have a pump, this basal insulin coverage would be achieved by using different types of insulin at different times throughout the day. An endocrinologist would be the one to prescribe these. There have been times, however, that strenuous exercises have raised my blood glucose. This confirms the importance of always having the glucometer at hand.

I've also learned to check my blood glucose whenever I'm out in the sun for extended periods. Even if I'm just walking outside, the heat can have an effect on my glucose. One summer, we went to Disney World in July. It was hot and humid, and we were walking a lot. I checked my blood glucose constantly, almost every hour. The effect of being under the hot sun and all that walking was dramatic! My blood glucose was pretty low most of my vacation time and I had to drastically reduce the amount of insulin that I was taking every day. It was a change for me and I had to adjust.

Speaking of adjustments, I've had to periodically adjust my treatment of my diabetes because being a woman plays a big role in the highs and lows; hormones can be our worst enemy. In my case, my glucose numbers were very different during the first week of my menses compared to the other three weeks. If one is going through menopause, the roller coaster is even worse. If one is pregnant, one really, really needs to constantly check one's blood glucose. The natural ups and downs during one's pregnancy plus being a PWD woman really complicates things. I remember during my first pregnancy, I was amazed at how much insulin I needed to cover 8 ounces of orange juice. You would have thought I was having a meal!

Whenever possible, wash your hands or use alcohol swabs to clean your fingers before you check your blood glucose. Believe it or not, substances on your fingers could give you numbers that may be off by 40 points. It's happened to me plenty of times: I feel low, check my blood glucose, and find that I have a decent number. I keep feeling low, check again, and the number is higher. Something is clearly not right. I wash my hands, check my blood glucose again, and I've gone down 40 points from the first reading!

If you're wondering why I would check my blood glucose if I feel low, there is a simple answer: there are times where I feel tired, sluggish, and weak, then check my blood glucose only to find that I'm actually experiencing a *high*. Low or high, you definitely want to treat an accurate number. As long as you are mentally and physically able, it is important to always try to check your blood glucose *before* treating yourself. This is important because diabetes is very unpredictable. I always test my blood glucose as soon as I suspect I may be having a low or a high.

Once I've confirmed a low or a high, I immediately need to treat it. One thing I will suggest is don't use candy as a way of treating a low. Yes, candy will raise your glucose, but it will take longer because foods that have fat slow down the process of raising the blood glucose. When having a low, fast results are essential. Every PWD should at least know about what is called a Glucagon Emergency Kit. A Glucagon Emergency Kit is not for everyone, but every PWD should know what it is and discuss it with their physician. We will discuss this in detail in a later chapter.

Treating a high is just as important as treating a low. I cannot wait until I get home to treat a high. No, it needs to be treated the moment I become aware of it, just like when I become aware of a low. Remember, the consequences of a high may not always be visible or felt immediately; however, if I am consistently high, the consequences are horrific. The way I prepare myself to treat my highs is by always carrying my form of treatment with me everywhere I go. As previously mentioned, my form of treatment is insulin. How you treat a high glucose number has to be a discussion you and your physician have. There's a numerical formula called the insulin sensitivity factor, which determines how many points in mg/dl your blood glucose levels will drop for each unit of insulin taken. This term is also known as the "correction factor" because I will use this formula to fix a high if needed. If you are someone living with T1D and don't know your sensitivity factor, you need to ask your healthcare provider to explain this term to you and to work with you to get a numerical formula[17] that will work for you. The process to determine your correction factor is complicated and I would not advise anyone to do this on their own.

While the above is about how to deal with highs and lows while actively experiencing them, there are a lot of other things you can do to decrease and/or prevent highs and lows, including but not limited to:

Technology: If you have a continuous glucose monitor, be sure to calibrate it during its course. Most continuous glucose monitors last about 10 days on you. They are good and life saving, but not always accurate. If you feel low and your continuous glucose monitor does not say that, test your blood glucose. On a different note, if you are following your every day routine and nothing major has changed and your blood glucose is higher than normal, check your insulin pump and check the date on your insulin. Something might not be right. If you feel you are having trouble with the accuracy of your technology, REPORT IT to their companies. These companies are continuously looking to improve our lives and they want to know if something is not working well, which leads me to the next important thing.

Advocate: You should be your best advocate. If you see that your numbers are not where they are supposed to be, see your doctor. Ask to see a nutritionist and arm yourself by learning as much as possible about how to treat your diabetes. If you don't have health insurance, there are lots of books at the library that can help you understand diabetes. Keep in mind that despite what any book tells you (including this one), everyone's diabetes is different; your diabetes is your disease and you must be the one in charge of it. And only you will come to know how your diabetes affects you and how everything you do affects your diabetes. For example, any other non-diabetes related medications you may be on can affect your glucose numbers. If this happens, you need to work with your endocrinologist and the provider that prescribed you that medication to see how this situation should be addressed.

Be part of a team: When at all possible and if you have medical insurance, have a team of doctors that can help you and educate you. You should have at least an endocrinologist, a diabetes educator, a dietician, an eye doctor, and a foot doctor. If you have other health conditions, you may need to have more members on your team. For example, if you have heart conditions, you need a cardiologist, and so on.

Have goals: Set healthy goals for your diabetes. Setting these healthy goals helps me stay focused and in line. Here are some examples of my goals:

- My A1C should be under 7.00

- My cholesterol level should be[18]:

    o LDL Cholesterol: Less than 100 mg/dL
    o HDL Cholesterol: Greater than 40 mg/dL
    o Triglycerides: Less than 150 mg/dL

- My kidney functions should remain normal
- The level of protein in my urine should remain normal

And the list of goals can go on and on and on. You may say, "What is so special about my cholesterol, shouldn't everyone's cholesterol remain healthy? Shouldn't everyone's kidneys always function properly?" The answer is YES; however, if I am having difficulty managing my diabetes, it will affect my health on so many levels, and in such ugly and unhealthy ways.

Treat your diabetes like a child: Your diabetes needs YOU (the parent) to take care of it. It needs discipline, structure, and consistency. Like a child, your diabetes requires regular, specific health checks[19] that are vital to its care.

Forgive yourself: If you fall off the wagon, it's okay. Forgive yourself and get right back on it. To this day, I still fall off the wagon more often than I would like to admit. Remember that you are human, always be kind to yourself.

Educate your family: Your loved ones need to be educated as to how serious diabetes is and how they can be part of your treatment team by being supportive and by knowing how to help you if you ever find yourself in an extreme low or an extreme high. For example, when my boys were younger, I would tell them, "If mommy doesn't wake up, you call daddy or 911 if daddy isn't home." Explain to your children that if they ever find themselves in a situation like this, they need to inform the caller or the people around them that, "My mom/dad has diabetes." Role play with the kids, they need to know exactly what to say and what to do. Before I had the technology that I have now, I would tell my husband, "Honey, if you see me struggling to wake up in the mornings when I'm supposed to be up and getting ready to go to work, please wake me up and ask me to check my glucose."

At work: If you work, let your co-workers know that you are a PWD. In your workspace, keep your emergency contacts handy and let a few people know where this information is. For example, I was blessed (in many ways) to work at a school for a great number of years. My school nurse knew of my diabetes and had all my emergency contacts. My co-workers also knew of my diabetes.

Do not keep your diabetes a secret: A PWD, no matter what type, should always wear a medical bracelet. In the past few years, these have become very fashionable. I recommend owning more than one because these can get lost. Also, keep a card in your wallet or in your car. I share this with you because for me, when I was first diagnosed with diabetes, I was ashamed and embarrassed. It took me a while to overcome these feelings and recognize the fact that letting those around me know that I am a person with T1D could one day save my life.

If you go to the gym, yoga, women's groups, church groups, etc., do not keep your diabetes a secret. You'll be surprised how many others may be living with diabetes or have a close person in their life that is a PWD. Do not be ashamed of being a PWD. Being ashamed of one's diabetes will not help you in any way. Acceptance is one of the key first steps when living with diabetes. The sooner you accept the fact that you are a PWD, that you are special, that you are unique, the sooner you will embrace your treatment plan. Also keep in mind that your diabetes treatment is not found in a perfect, numerical formula. Its treatment is not found in a chart according to your weight. Its treatment is not a "one size fits all" kind of treatment. Its treatment also does not have an end date.

So, go ahead, give it a name and a gender if you wish because diabetes will be right there with you until the end, as faithful as anyone could ever be.

Chapter XI: Acceptance Is The Hardest Thing

I have now been living with diabetes for over 30 years. The question is: have I accepted my diabetes? The answer to that question could be a book in itself. Receiving the diagnosis of diabetes is life-changing. A PWD can honestly go through the five stages of grief[20]. The five stages are denial, anger, bargaining, depression, and acceptance. Although getting a diagnosis of diabetes is not losing a loved one, it's definitely a loss and a huge change. It's the loss of how I used to live my life and of all the things I used to love to eat that I now can't or shouldn't eat.

- Denial may sound like, " I can't possibly have diabetes. Look at me, I'm healthy."
- Anger may sound like, "Why me? What did I do to deserve this?'

- Bargaining may sound like, "If I give myself extra insulin, I can have that piece of pie."

- Depression may sound like, "I hate my life. Life is not fair, nothing good can come out of this."

- Acceptance: … Let's talk about acceptance.

I will begin by saying that acceptance is the hardest thing. When it comes to diabetes, acceptance is not just being able to say, "Yes, my name is Marie and I have diabetes." No, it is much more than that. When it comes to acceptance, it means realizing that being a PWD means being unique, being different, and also being somewhat okay with this. Acceptance also means that one is willing to make a lifestyle change. It means that one is willing to say, "No, thank you," more often than, "Sure, I would love that."

To me, accepting my diabetes starts within me *every single day*. Unfortunately, there are days that I forget I'm a PWD; however, for the most part, I accept the fact that I live with diabetes every day of my life. Every morning when I wake up, I grab my insulin pump and continuous glucose monitor from under my pillow, and take them with me to the bathroom, that's acceptance. The morning when I choose to have a healthy breakfast rather than a bagel with cream cheese (believe me, I would prefer the latter,) that's acceptance. Every time that I wake up in the middle of the night to go to the bathroom and first look at my continuous glucose monitor, that's acceptance. Every time I have my blood drawn to get my A1C, cholesterol, and other important tests, then anxiously wait to see what my numbers are, that's acceptance. Every time I measure my food and count how many grapes I will eat, that's acceptance. Prior to the technology I have today, every time I did math in my head before each meal because the amount of carbohydrates determined the amount of insulin needed, that was acceptance. When using syringes, every time I had to inject my insulin and I looked for a new spot on my body, one without a mark, that was acceptance.

Acceptance is not always easy or graceful. Every time I check my glucose and my number is extremely high and I curse out loud with frustration and wonder why, then realize I forgot to take my insulin after my last meal, so I rush to remedy that number, that's acceptance with frustration. Every time I check my glucose and I have a high number that I can't explain and am almost in tears with frustration and I say how much I hate being a PWD, once again, that's acceptance with frustration. Every time I'm going somewhere special, let's say a wedding, and I struggle with where I'm going to carry my glucometer, my insulin pump, my continuous glucose monitor, my phone, and GOD forbid I forget my glucose tablets, that's acceptance. Every time I go to the gym or just want to go for a walk in my neighborhood and I have to check my glucose and pack my fanny bag just to go around the block with my dog, that's acceptance. Again, my acceptance of my diabetes happens every second of my life. Sometimes that acceptance may not be happy, but it is there.

Being a PWD also means that I am willing to make permanent changes. These permanent changes will not only be in my diet, but also in my lifestyle. Like I said before, the days of only carrying just my wallet and money are over. If a PWD drinks regular soda, they should really stop that. To this day, I still remember when I had my first diet soda drink; it was a gross experience. On the other side of the coin, I also remember the day I was accidentally given a glass of regular soda after drinking diet soda for months. It was also a gross experience. I instantly spat out the soda because my taste buds had truly changed. That was acceptance and reminded me that change is always possible. With that in mind, years later, I stopped drinking diet soda for good! That's acceptance. In a nutshell, I have to live differently than everyone else! This is the biggest challenge a newly-diagnosed PWD has to embrace. The reality is that winning this challenge does not happen overnight. It all depends on the individual but it will *always* be a challenge.

To me, diabetes is truly a full-time job. Being a PWD is living with diabetes 24/7 for the rest of that individual's life. There are no breaks, no vacations, no respite. In very simple terms, being a PWD means that one's body is not able to handle food the proper way; therefore, food is a huge curse for a PWD. For a PWD, food can be like poison if they don't make many permanent and serious changes. As a society, we are accustomed to viewing food as comfort. We are conditioned to eat food to feel happy. Food has been there to comfort us when we feel stressed. Food makes us feel better when we are sad. Food is a safety blanket for most people, me included. Food has been like medicine for many. Unfortunately, it's not always the best medicine for people living with diabetes. I know of many occasions when I've had a rough day and I crave certain types of food. Usually these foods are not on the good list for me. At the same time, we all need food to survive. It is the biggest catch 22 for any person living with diabetes. Accepting one's diabetes diagnosis means that one is willing to see food as fuel rather than as comfort, pleasurable, or as a security blanket *more often than not*. Getting to this realization can not only be difficult, it can also be painful, discouraging, very frustrating, and at times, it will feel like it is a completely impossible task.

Lastly, the key thing to remember is that before anyone ever becomes a Person With Diabetes, one is and always will be human first. Once that diagnosis is made, however, one must never, ever, ever forget that one is now a *human being living with diabetes*. Never forget that you are unique. Never forget that you need to live a different lifestyle compared to those that are not living with diabetes. Also remember that when you choose to make an exception with food every now and then, you have to be very, very cautious.

And you must know there will be serious consequences for constantly "forgetting" that you are a PWD.

If I ever wondered what being part of an experiment would be like, the day I was given the diagnosis of T1D was the day I automatically entered my own life-long experiment. Yes, "life-long experiment." One thing every person with diabetes must know and always remember is that one's treatment is not written in stone. My life-long experiment has required me to do some documentation and analysis to determine how foods affect me. I've created sheets, both handwritten and on the computer, where I would document what and how much I was eating, the amount of carbs, and my glucose numbers before and after eating. This made it easy for me to learn how the meals I ate affected my blood glucose numbers. There was a time that I decided to eat the same type of meals for an entire 30 days. For these 30 days, I ate the same breakfast, lunch, and dinner. I don't remember what my breakfasts and lunches were but my dinners were grilled salmon and steamed vegetables. What did I learn? I learned that if I stick to the foods that I know work for me, I reduce the unpredictability of my diabetes. I learned that being spontaneous when I go out to dinner is not always as extravagant as it sounds for someone like me. I'm better off having that salad with salmon, dressing on the side, skip the cranberries and the candied walnuts. It is very frustrating not being able to try new things without having to worry. Okay, frustrating is too nice of a word. It's beyond frustrating and is really annoying! But in the end, it turns out to be a good choice. If I ever do choose to be spontaneous, I am vigilant in checking my blood glucose numbers and adjust my insulin as needed. I have learned that if I am adventurous or spontaneous, it's best if I do it during my early meals (breakfast or lunch.) This way, I don't spend my night struggling with highs or lows because I might have miscalculated my insulin dose. Planning ahead like this, that's acceptance.

Also, please know that if your doctor tells you to do x, y and z, three times a day, this may not be the same recommendation three months or a year later. Many aspects of life will affect one's diabetes. For example, if I get sick, I need a "sick treatment plan". If I am on vacation, I may need to adjust my treatment plan depending on the type of vacation. When I was pregnant, I definitely needed a different treatment plan. As I get older, I see my needs changing. Most importantly, these changes will differ from person to person. The one and only way to know when one needs to change their treatment plan is to constantly check one's blood glucose and to have an active medical team.

Lastly, please remember acceptance will not come easy and as a person living with diabetes, every day is a new day. As described in a previous chapter, I have hope that my diabetes will be successful in life. Besides hope, I also have perseverance. Yes, as someone living with T1D, I have to try my hardest and I've come to find out that my hardest is just starting over every single day of my life. Whenever I wake up with a number I cannot explain, I remind myself that every day is a new day for me.

Chapter XII: The World Does Not Think Like a PWD

My youngest son at age 8 was very well aware that food had to be eaten in portions, as was my oldest son when he was 13 years old. It was music to my ears when I would hear the two of them ask, "Mom, how much of this can I eat?" It was even better when I would reply by asking my 13-year-old son how many calories and carbohydrates were in each serving, and he was able to look at the label and tell me. One day, my youngest son told me that I should open up a restaurant where only healthy food is sold. He was a bit surprised at my answer: "You know, I have thought about that myself, but I'm afraid not many people will go to it." Very confused, he asked why I thought that and I said, "Well, the world does not think like mommy." What I really wanted to say was, "The world does not think like people who live with diabetes!"

How do we know the world does not think like a PWD? Let's look at something as simple as going out to eat.

When you go to a restaurant, the menu you are given very seldom has a breakdown of the calories and/or carbohydrates for each meal. The menu also does not tell you how many servings you are eating. Is it one serving of meat, two servings of vegetables, and one serving of bread for this meal? This calculation is something a PWD will have to do on their own and, most of the time, we find ourselves playing the guessing game. Thankfully, a lot of restaurants will now have this nutritional information on their website, but you obviously have to take the time to seek out this information. Let me make it known that I myself love going out to dinner but if this nutritional information was readily available on every restaurant's menu, I would think twice about my meal choice.

Although I am a big fan of going out to dinner, I was shocked to see how high in calories my "healthy" meals were when I discovered this information online. Let's consider fish with spinach, is this harmless and healthy? If you make it at home, the answer is yes but this dish at a restaurant can have up to or more than 500 calories. Why? Oils, butter, sauces, everything that may add flavor will change the meal. So if you don't have access to this nutritional information at your favorite restaurant, be sure to always ask how your meal is made, including what oils, sauces, and ingredients are in it. Remember, the entire world does not live with diabetes, nor is it concerned about gaining too much weight, thus it does not think like a PWD.

Once someone is diagnosed as a PWD, they will need to constantly experiment with food. For example, there used to be this one particular restaurant in my neighborhood that had the best bread rolls. Even though I had been to this restaurant and had these rolls many times, I had a very hard time getting the insulin ratio right, and I had a very hard time resisting them. This is what I call "my human moment" and at that time, I would give myself the grace to still enjoy these rolls. It can be very frustrating to eat something multiple times but the insulin ratio can vary. So how did I deal with this? First, I didn't eat them every day. Second, I used to take the inside of the bread roll out and enjoy the rest of it. Third, I didn't get down on myself if the insulin ratio didn't work on a given occasion.

I also accepted the fact that these bread rolls had to be added to my "really should not eat or drink this" list. Regular soda falls on that list, and should for any PWD. White rice is also now on that list because my body has a hard time processing it and I just don't think it's worth the hassle, meaning the hassle of starting with a good glucose number prior to eating it, then having to deal with a high number three hours later despite the adjustments I might've made. There are also certain foods that I feel there isn't enough insulin in the world to cover them (waffles fall under that category for me.) I must admit, there are times when I make exceptions for these types of food. For example, when I went to Puerto Rico one hot summer after 11 years of being in the States and I had the privilege of having Mom's homemade traditional Puerto Rican foods like arroz con gandules and tostones, I couldn't say no. Actually, I didn't *want* to say no, so I made an exception!

Since our society does not think like a PWD, what can a PWD do? Again, think of yourself as being part of a "life-long experiment." The first thing you need to do is master the art of knowing what carbohydrates do to your blood glucose. Whether you are newly diagnosed with diabetes or not, you should always experiment with your food with your doctor's guidance. Remember to check your blood glucose before eating and two hours after eating. Another technique I've used is to eat the same type of food a few times, always making note of what my blood glucose was before I ate and two hours after. For example, let's say your favorite meal at a restaurant is one roll dipped in olive oil with garlic and two slices of pizza. Although you may have the nutritional information for this meal, your carb ratio may not work; therefore, you should experiment with this same menu more than once to see how this meal affects your blood glucose and how much insulin you need each time. Write down your before and after numbers so that you remember them. There are some very sophisticated glucometers out there that can store a lot of data for you. If you take pills, see how this meal affects you and keep track of that so you can determine what to eat and what not to eat. Regardless of your treatment, remember to *always* consult with your medical team prior to experimenting.

Another time you may see how our society does not think like a PWD is when you go to a social gathering. Unless the person hosting the gathering has diabetes, chances are they won't know how many carbohydrates are in each dish. Why? Because, unless the host is living with diabetes, they are most likely not too concerned about how many carbohydrates a meal has. Consider it a blessing if they happen to have sugar substitutes for your coffee or tea. You may also hear comments like, "Oh, nothing in today's meal has sugar, so you can eat as much as you can," or "Oh, this dessert is made with artificial sugar, so you can eat as much as you'd like." If they see you measuring your food, you may get comments like, "Oh, my food is healthy and it won't raise your sugar." Sometimes I feel people may get offended if they see that you brought a food item for yourself or if they see that you are measuring what you eat of their food. Again, I tell you our society does not think like a PWD. How have I dealt with people's comments? Honestly, I try to shrug them off. I have come to learn that people don't really care to hear the truth about food. I only go into details if people genuinely ask me to explain the what, why, and how.

Sadly, diabetes can affect anyone. Diabetes does not pick and choose their victims. Diabetes affects children, teens, adults, even animals. If a school-aged child living with diabetes eats food from their school menu, that menu most likely will not have their food broken down into how many carbohydrates each meal has. However, under the Americans with Disabilities Act and the Rehabilitation Act, any student with diabetes has rights to certain accommodations[21]. This is when parents and/or caretakers have to advocate and work with the school system to get their child's needs met.

Recently, fast food restaurants have begun to provide important information about each meal: carbohydrates, calories, fat, and much more. Of course, fast food is not the type of food a PWD should be eating. If someone living with diabetes makes the choice to eat fast food, they must remember to count their carbohydrates. There are small pocket books that will tell you critical information on most types of food. I am a "recovered junk food eater." At the time in my life when I was a junk food eater, fast food restaurants were not providing this information so I kept my pocket carb counter book on me so that I could determine the correct amount of insulin. Again, you may find the needed information for a fast food restaurant, but you won't find it at your town's annual fair when you purchase food from there.

Our society does not understand that a diet for someone living with diabetes does not equate to a diet without sugar. As advanced as our society can be, it still does not seem to understand that carbohydrates become sugar. Although ½ cup of white rice does not have sugar, it will turn into sugar in your body. I feel that our society is slowly accepting the fact that brown rice is much healthier, and more healthy choices are becoming widely available, but there's a lot more work to be done. I have dreams and hopes that one day, hopefully sooner rather than later, our society will provide this critical information for food at all places. I must say that our society is becoming much more health conscious, but as a society, we have a long way to go. It is hard to live in a society that is not thinking of those living with diabetes. But there are a few things that you can do to make things easier for you as a PWD. Here are a few tips that have helped me along the way:

- If you use sugar substitutes, always carry some with you. Have some at the office, in your supply bag, in your car, your partner's car, just about anywhere.

- There are plenty of carbohydrate counter books that are small enough to fit anywhere and have a ton of information. You can also find carb counter apps to download to your smartphone. This way, if you go to a restaurant or eat at a social gathering, you can calculate on your own how many carbohydrates your meal may have. If math is not your strength, carry a small calculator with you if you don't have your cell phone with you.

- If you like drinks with substitute sweeteners, you can find diet sodas anywhere. If you don't drink diet soda and you are not a fan of water, there are plenty of powdered sugar-free drink mixes that come in carry-on size for your convenience.

- If you are going to someone's house, offer to bring a dish or two that are suited for you. Bring enough to share with everyone and even if your dish is not the hit of the gathering, at least you know what you are eating.

- Always carry your medication with you, whatever this may be. If you are on an insulin pump, always carry all that you need to switch your pump in case it malfunctions on you. Think of it as gasoline for your car. You wouldn't go anywhere if your car runs out of gas, right? My rule is I can't go anywhere if I don't have my insulin, my delivery system, and my glucometer.

- It is also critical to carry something that will raise your sugar in a safe manner. I carry glucose tablets in my car, my husband's car, and in my purse. I have a glucagon kit with me at all times. As I stated in earlier chapters, glucagon is a hormone that is produced by the body in those who don't have diabetes to raise their blood glucose levels. Glucagon kits are available by prescription to PWDs, particularly to those living with T1D or who use insulin. They have several kinds of glucagon kits on the market and they are lifesavers.[22] If you don't have one or don't know what a glucagon kit is, talk to your healthcare provider about this and your provider will tell you whether or not you should have one. In twenty plus years, I've been low more times than I would like to admit to and I have mostly used my glucose tablets and/or juice to raise my sugar. I have, however, used the glucagon kit a total of three times because I wasn't able to raise my blood glucose quickly enough and I was afraid I was going to pass out.

- This one was extreme for me, but I've found that it's helped me live a healthier life: I made the decision to stop eating meat (beef, pork and poultry) and decided to add fish into my diet. I previously tried eating vegetables for breakfast because I learned that my body is very sensitive to carbs in the morning. This was no easy task, I must say! I later switched to a very high protein/low carb breakfast instead.

- Last, but not least, please remember that you are unique and very special, but most of all, you must be the one in charge of your body and your health, and you should always and forever expect the BEST for your diabetes!

Although the world does not think like a PWD; diabetes happens to be the seventh leading cause of death in this country. Millions of individuals in the US had diabetes in

2018 (to be more accurate, that was about 34.2 million people) these included diagnosed or undiagnosed.[23] [24] Although the world does not think like a PWD; diabetes is a disability under the Americans with Disabilities Act and the Rehabilitation Act. It is also referred to as an "invisible disability"; one should never be discriminated against due to their diabetes![25].

Chapter XIII: My Journey With Diabetes

I began my journey as a woman living with diabetes the day I was diagnosed with it. It has been a journey with ups and downs. A journey with rocky mountains and scary cliffs. A journey full of frustration, anger, sadness, and many painful moments. It has also been full of intriguing moments with all kinds of surprises. It has been full of many learning experiences and opportunities to improve not only my health and well-being, but also the well-being of my loved ones. Nevertheless, I can honestly say that I've tried very, very hard to keep it a positive experience. I repeat, I have *tried* very, very hard to keep it a positive experience.

How can I see positivity in a disease one may ask? For me, becoming a PWD was a blessing in disguise. I was a heavy-duty junk food fan and diabetes forced me to have a healthier lifestyle. If you had asked me thirty years ago if I thought I would ever have the eating habits that I currently have, I would have told you that was impossible! I'm here to tell you that one's success with diabetes depends a lot on one's own willingness to change and one's level of acceptance of the fact that they have diabetes. Let me remind you that this acceptance and willingness to change did not happen overnight for me. It took me seeing my mom, who did not have diabetes, struggle with her own health.

The year 2013 brought a whole different perspective to me in terms of health, life, death, and the future as one ages with health issues. On December 31, 2012, my dearest mom underwent an open-heart surgery at the age of 82. As my sister and I flew over the Atlantic Ocean and spent New Year's Eve in the air for the first time in our lives, we waited and prayed for our mom's well-being. We knew her surgery would be high risk, but we never, ever expected what was to come. As my sister and I arrived at her bedside, we found our mom with two incisions: one to her chest and a leg-length incision to her right leg where they had taken a vein to fix her heart's condition.

As I watched our 83 year old mother, who had several health struggles but had never been diagnosed with diabetes despite the family history of type 2 diabetes, I bewilderedly and ironically saw her suffer physical consequences that I would have expected of someone with diabetes. My mom's kidneys shut down on her and I stood next to her as she went through a treatment of dialysis. I watched my fire-strong mom unable to get out of the bed, or put one foot in front of the other. Despite the cardiologist's claims that her heart was now new after surgery, my mom's heart was so weak that it was not able to pump enough blood and oxygen to her lower extremities. As a result, her right foot was the color of an eggplant and her leg-length incision never healed 100%. Part of the lower part of her wound opened and I was able to see the inside of her leg. It was the most uncivilized thing I had ever seen, yet I could not believe I was actually seeing this. Her open wound remained open and she caught sepsis and eventually died. All of this happened in 66 days, from going into the hospital until the moment she died. It should be noted that she was being treated at a mediocre hospital and I will never know if her being at a better hospital would have made a difference.

After watching my Mom's health quickly deteriorate and dying 66 days later, I once again said to myself, "I really need to take care of my health." I honestly feel that I do an okay job caring for my diabetes and health, but I saw my Mom's death as another awakening moment, one in which I realized how fragile life truly is. Sadly, I have heard people who know diabetes is in their genes say, "Well, why bother trying to prevent it? I'm doomed to have diabetes anyway." That is not a good attitude to have. The one thing you can know for sure if you have diabetes in your genes is that you are *at risk* of getting diabetes, it is not necessarily guaranteed. Type 1 continues to be a mystery to science and I pray science can unlock this mystery in my lifetime. And I think we can all agree that living a healthy lifestyle can lead to good things.

I also see my diabetes as a blessing because the work that I have done and the education I have gotten from it has enabled me to teach my children how to take care of their bodies and what eating healthy can look like. I must say, it is not an easy battle and I did not earn the title of "Food Patrol" from my husband without a lot of work. But when my children were young and I would see them get cookies out of the pantry, read the food label, and just have one serving rather than eating until they were full, I saw my diabetes as a blessing. When I heard them say, "Oh, I can't have cookies again because I already had cookies today," I saw my diabetes as a blessing. I taught them how important it is to eat healthy, exercise, and maintain a healthy weight. I pray that my struggles and my journey are a good lesson to them and that they continue to learn how to lead healthy lives. Today, they are 22 and 17 years old and I am very proud of their discipline with food.

As someone who lives with diabetes, I still have lots of changes to embrace but as I've said before, every day is a new day. Every day when I wake up, I pray and hope to have a good day. Every day is a new opportunity for me to make things work in a positive way. Every day I struggle to do well, to make good choices, to have great numbers. Whenever I have an "out of range glucose day," it's frustrating and discouraging, but all I can do is start all over again.

In my journey, I've learned to forgive myself. I've learned to try new foods I would have never eaten before, like avocados. I've learned that change can be a good thing. I've learned that I'm always working on my diabetes and I'm always learning. I've also learned that I know myself better than anyone else. I've learned that the older I get, my goals related to my diabetes become more challenging and much more difficult to achieve. In spite of that and, despite my age and how old my diabetes is, I still have high expectations for my first child and I must expect the best of her.

There are a few other things I've learned in my journey that I would like to share with you:

1. If you have diabetes, life insurance companies don't want to insure you and if they do, your premiums are very, very high.

2. Medical insurance can often become an obstacle for you; however, you as the PWD need to be your best advocate.

3. You can get a lot of your supplies for free. Ask your doctor, he/she may be able to guide you in the right direction.

4. I've learned that yes, just like at the doctor's office, it is important to wash your hands before you prick your finger and test your glucose. You would be amazed at the things you may get on your fingers throughout the day and how these things can affect your readings.

5. I've learned that if I change my insulin bottle every four weeks, I see better results.

6. I've learned that exercise can be the most natural treatment for people with diabetes and there are certain exercises that, if I do them after a meal, allow me to use less insulin and still end up with a good number two hours later (this is my experience, everyone is different and should always consult with their medical team.)

7. I've learned that my dogs can tell when my glucose is low and will go out of their way to tell me. This has happened to me multiple times before I got my continuous glucose monitor. Two of my labrador retrievers went out of their way to wake me up from low glucose levels. My dogs were not trained as support dogs, but there are dogs that are trained to be support dogs who can assist a PWD[26].

8. I've learned that my glucose rises a lot quicker in the morning when I rush out the door without eating.

9. I've learned that my diabetes is very alive and active while I'm sleeping. It does not sleep!

10. I've learned that, as a PWD, I must do extra preparation when a natural disaster may occur. Natural disasters like tornadoes, hurricanes, and serious storms can force you out of your home. If you look at your diabetes like your child, that will make it easier to think of it during such a chaotic time. If you have ample time to plan ahead before needing to leave your home, you must be sure to have enough diabetes supplies to cover for that time away from home. If the natural disaster does not give you ample time to plan ahead, it is critical to have your doctor's name and phone number, as well as your pharmacy's contact information handy, in addition to taking what supplies you can. When natural disasters occur, this is when it's most critical that you are wearing a medical ID.

I could keep on adding and adding to this list, but this book would have taken longer to get to you. If you have diabetes, then you know once someone is diagnosed as a PWD, they automatically enter into a very unique journey that never ends. Just the basics of caring for one's diabetes can exhaust anyone, but it is a journey worth taking on. My diabetes and caring for her has become a life-long journey. If you are PWD, I'm sure you, as well as I, don't want this journey to end anytime soon. I want this journey to last for a very long time. I also want to enjoy this journey, be happy for most of it, and feel alive and healthy along the way.

EPILOGUE

Writing this book has been a tremendous journey and a *long* process! I began writing when my children were much younger. Since then, I went from using insulin and syringes as my mode of treatment to switching to an insulin pump. I then decided to go back to syringes, to then quickly go back to an insulin pump. In 2013, I came to discover one of the best instruments of today's technology that I can honestly say makes diabetes somewhat manageable: a continuous glucose monitor. My continuous glucose monitor gives me a blood glucose reading at all times.

Technology has become a great part of my life with my T1D and because of the technology I have today, I don't have to test my blood glucose as often as I used to when I didn't have this technology. Today, everywhere I go (and I mean everywhere, including the bathroom,) I bring three devices with me: my insulin pump, my continuous glucose monitor, and my cell phone. Both my insulin pump and my continuous glucose monitor can communicate with my smartphone. Having this technology makes life a bit easier in many ways. I recognize that I am privileged to have good health insurance that allows me to have this technology and to be able to switch doctors when the fit wasn't right. If you don't have this privilege, please continue to be your best and loudest advocate. Talk to your local and state representatives, join a movement of change that may already exist, ask your doctors for ways of getting free diabetes supplies. It's not going to hurt you to ask.

Although I have my continuous glucose monitor with me at all times, I still need to test my blood glucose to calibrate my continuous glucose monitor. The continuous glucose monitor is not accurate 100% of the time, but it's pretty close more often than not. This technology has saved my life in instances when I don't feel my extreme lows, particularly in my sleep. This device will beep/vibrate and wake me or my husband up in the middle of the night, alerting me to a low or a high. These devices have to be within a certain distance from me and I don't go anywhere without them. I sleep with my insulin pump and continuous glucose monitor under my pillow or next to it. I also sleep with a juice box or glucose tablets within arm's reach. Although I am not physically connected to these devices by wires, I am attached to them. If I go out of the required distance range, I will lose the connection and not be able to get my blood glucose reading or give myself a bolus.

The experience of watching my mother's health decline after her surgery in 2013 made me wonder what will become of me and my diabetes as I get older. Will I be able to take care of my health? Will I be able to take care of my diabetes, or as I like to call her, my daughter? Would I be able to manage the technology I have today twenty years from now? How about when I'm 80? My hope is that the answer is yes, I will. I don't have a crystal ball, nor can I see what lies ahead in my future. But I do know that what I do today with my health, how I treat it, how I care for it, how I eat, how much or how little I exercise, and how I work to maintain a healthy weight will affect my future. All I know is that today, I need to continue to do what I know is best for me.

Since the day I started writing this book, I have made many changes. I stopped eating meat. I stopped drinking soda (with the exception of ginger ale when my stomach has been upset.) I welcome technology into my mode of treatment for my diabetes. I have changed my endocrinologist multiple times, looking for the one I am happy with today. As for my general health providers, I switched to a naturopathic practice, including an MD that follows their views. I went from having young children to being menopausal. Boy, has that been a challenge to my diabetes! I developed another autoimmune disease (hypothyroidism) and most recently, I have been diagnosed with mild nonproliferative retinopathy. I now do yoga and I meditate. I've heard more times than I would like to count, "Oh yes, people with diabetes are prone to get that and that and the other."

I do not have a crystal ball! But I do have the power to make healthy choices every day of my life. I do have the power to say, "No, thank you," more often than not. I may not be able to predict my future, but I can help and contribute to a brighter future with diabetes, and that is my goal. My goal is to live as healthy as I possibly can. When I die, I want my grave to at least say, *~She died trying~*.

Last but not least, I have a very strong support system. My husband and my children (all 4 of them) are very supportive of me. I also have supportive family members, supportive friends, and a supportive work environment. I also have a very strong faith in a higher power. My faith (which I am grateful to my mom for instilling in me) has always been a source of strength to me. For all of this, I am forever grateful!

If you are someone living with diabetes and just finished reading this book, whether you are type 1 or type 2, your health is worth taking care of. I know caring for diabetes can be extremely draining, exhausting, and overwhelming, and it can have a serious impact on your mental health. Please take care of your health and seek support, both physically and emotionally. Although you are the one who can best care for your diabetes, you do not need to do this alone, nor should you ever try to go on this journey alone. If it helps, my affirmations are as follows: Stay Strong, Never Stop Praying, Every Day is a New Day. As you can see, taking care of one's diabetes, *It's not just about the sugar*. It is very complicated, to say the least.

May the world become a better place for all and may science find a cure for diabetes!

Marie A.C. Cortez, LCSW (M.A.C.C.)

ACKNOWLEDGMENTS

I want to thank my stepdaughter Stephanie A. Cortez for the countless times she read this book and edited it. Your time, dedication and your work is ***greatly appreciated.*** I could not have done this without you

Notes

1. Mike Hoskins, "Words Matter: The Debate Over 'Diabetic' vs. 'Person with Diabetes'," Healthline, March 9, 2021, https://www.healthline.com/diabetesmine/the-word-diabetic#Why-diabetic-can-be-offensive.

2. Maria Muccioli, "The History of Diabetes: An Interactive Timeline," Diabetes Daily, July 1, 2021, https://www.diabetesdaily.com/learn-about-diabetes/basics/what-is-diabetes/the-history-of-diabetes-an-interactive-timeline.

3. "Monitoring Your Blood Sugar," Centers for Disease Control and Prevention, last reviewed August 10, 2021, https://www.cdc.gov/diabetes/managing/managing-blood-sugar/bloodglucosemonitoring.html.

4. "What is Type 1 Diabetes?," Centers for Disease Control and Prevention, last reviewed March 25, 2021, https://www.cdc.gov/diabetes/basics/what-is-type-1-diabetes.html.

5. Matthew Hoffman, "What are Autoimmune Disorders?," WebMD, June 22, 2020, https://www.webmd.com/a-to-z-guides/autoimmune-diseases.

6. "Learn the Genetics of Diabetes," American Diabetes Association, Copyright 1995-2021, https://www.diabetes.org/diabetes/genetics-diabetes.

7. Maria Muccioli, "The History of Diabetes: An Interactive Timeline," Diabetes Daily, July 1, 2021,

https://www.diabetesdaily.com/learn-about-diabetes/basics/what-is-diabetes/the-history-of-diabetes-an-interactive-timeline.

8. "Diabetes Basics," Centers for Disease Control and Prevention, last reviewed June 15, 2021, https://www.cdc.gov/diabetes/basics/index.html.

9. "Gestational Diabetes and a Healthy Baby? Yes.," American Diabetes Association, Copyright 1995-2021, https://www.diabetes.org/diabetes/gestational-diabetes.

10. "Hypoglycemia (Low Blood sugar)" American Diabetes Association,Copyright 1995–2021.

    https://diabetes.org/healthy-living/medication-treatments/blood-glucose-testing-and-control/hypoglycemia

11. Sarah Yang, "Baby's Checkup Schedule," The Bump, Updated March 2, 2017, https://www.thebump.com/a/new-baby-doctor-visit-checklist.

12. "Diabetes Report Card 2019," Centers for Disease Control and Prevention, last reviewed January 4, 2021, https://www.cdc.gov/diabetes/library/reports/reportcard.html.

13. "Hypoglycemia (Low Blood Glucose)," American Diabetes Association, Copyright 1995–2021, https://diabetes.org/healthy-living/medication-treatments/blood-glucose-testing-and-control/hypoglycemia

14. "Manage Blood Sugar," Centers for Disease
Control and Prevention, last reviewed April 28,
2021,
https://www.cdc.gov/diabetes/managing/manage-
blood-sugar.html.

15. "Eye Complications," American Diabetes
Association, Copyright 1995-2021,
https://diabetes.org/diabetes/complications/eye-
complications.

16. "Tight Control: Definition and Overview," Diabetes
Self-Management, June 16, 2006,
https://www.diabetesselfmanagement.com/diabetes-
resources/definitions/tight-
control/#:~:text=Tight%20control%20is%20a%20m
ethod,of%20preventing%20complications%20of%2
0diabetes.

17. "Determining Your Insulin Sensitivity Factor,"
Diabetes in Control, November 22, 2009,
http://www.diabetesincontrol.com/wp-
content/uploads/PDF/insulin_sensitivity_factor.pdf.

18. American Diabetes Association, "Dyslipidemia
Management in Adults with Diabetes," *Diabetes
Care* 27, no. suppl 1 (January 2004): s68-s71,
https://doi.org/10.2337/diacare.27.2007.S68

19. "Health Checks for People with Diabetes,"
American Diabetes Association, Copyright 1995-
2021, https://www.diabetes.org/diabetes/newly-
diagnosed/health-checks-people-with-diabetes.

20. Sandra Silva Casabianca, "Mourning and the 5
Stages of Grief," PsychCentral, February 11, 2021,

https://psychcentral.com/lib/the-5-stages-of-loss-and-grief#the-kubler-ross-model.

21. American Diabetes Association, "Know your rights, Safe at school"-1995-2022 https://www.diabetes.org/tools-support/know-your-rights/safe-at-school-state-laws

22. "Glucagon & Other Emergency Glucose Products," American Diabetes Association, Copyright 1995-2021, https://diabetes.org/healthy-living/medication-treatments/glucagon-other-emergency-glucose-products.

23. "Diabetes Data and Statistics," Centers for Disease Control and Prevention, last reviewed June 15, 2021, https://www.cdc.gov/diabetes/data/index.html.

24. "Diabetes 2019 Report Card," Centers for Disease Control and Prevention, 2020, https://www.cdc.gov/diabetes/pdfs/library/Diabetes-Report-Card-2019-508.pdf.

25. American Diabetes Association, "Is Diabetes a disability"-1995-2022 https://www.diabetes.org/tools-support/know-your-rights/discrimination/is-diabetes-a-disability#:~:text=Specifically%2C%20federal%20laws%2C%20such%20as,function%20of%20the%20endocrine%20system.

26. Sally Robertson, "Animals that can Detect Hypoglycemia," News Medical, last updated April 28, 2021, https://www.news-medical.net/health/Animals-That-Can-Detect-Hypoglycemia.aspx.

www.ingramcontent.com/pod-product-compliance
Lightning Source LLC
Chambersburg PA
CBHW062058270326
41931CB00013B/3133